GLUTEN-FREE & EASY

For Christine, thank you for your advice and for some great meals shared together
and for Ellie, a new recruit to the club.

First published in the United Kingdom in 2014 by
PAVILION BOOKS
10 Southcombe Street
London W14 0RA

An imprint of Anova Books Company Ltd

ISBN: 9781909108882

A CIP record for this book is available from the British Library

10 9 8 7 6 5 4 3 2 1

Reproduction by Dot Gradations, UK
Printed and bound by 1010 Printing international Ltd, China

Senior commissioning editor: Becca Spry
Assistant editor: Charlotte Selby
Art director and cover: Georgina Hewitt
Design: Maru Studio
Photography and styling: Liz and Max Haarala Hamilton
Food styling: Sara Lewis
Food styling assistant: Andrew Lewis
Step-by-step model: Georgie Wells
Editor: Maggie Ramsay
Production: Laura Brodie

Notes
The information in this book is not meant to replace advice from your doctor or other health
professionals. The author has included information that is to the best of her knowledge
correct and suitable for those on a gluten-free diet. Some ingredients may change, so always
check food packaging labels and information supplied and regularly updated by Coeliac UK
(www.coeliac.org.uk).

- Medium eggs are used.
- Some dishes contain nuts or nut derivatives. It is advisable for those with known allergic
  reactions or who may be potentially vulnerable – pregnant and nursing mothers, invalids, the
  elderly, babies and young children – to avoid these recipes.
- Microwave timings have been tested in a 750 watt oven: if your machine is more powerful,
  reduce the timings slightly; increase timings for a lower wattage oven.
- 🍽 indicates recipes that can be served cold the next day.

GLUTEN-FREE & EASY

OVER 80 SIMPLE RECIPES FOR THE GLUTEN INTOLERANT

SARA LEWIS

PAVILION

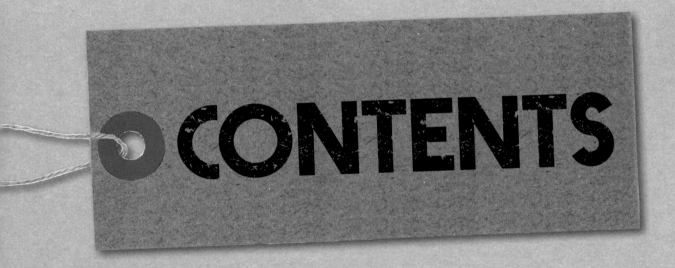

INTRODUCTION 6

PASTA,
GNOCCHI & NOODLES 16

FRIES 30

SAVOURY BAKES & ROASTS 46

PASTRY 62

BREAD 96

PUDDINGS 114

CAKES & COOKIES 130

INDEX 158

INTRODUCTION

You or your child, partner, relative or friend may have been advised by a doctor to go gluten-free. At first, this may seem a huge challenge, but gluten-free eating needn't mean missing out on the treats that others take for granted. Cakes, breads, pastries and puddings are all within reach. Gluten-free ingredients are now readily available from your local supermarket or health food shop (or online) and can be transformed into fab suppers to share with friends and family, from pasta dishes, pizzas and pancakes to light, moreish cakes and deliciously crumbly pies and tarts.

If you have just been diagnosed with coeliac disease, what you can buy and what you can cook may seem a little bewildering – you will need to avoid wheat, barley, rye, and any products containing them. If you have been diagnosed for a while you may feel as though you always cook the same dishes, week in week out. In this book you will find inspirational new recipes to eat alongside your old favourites, along with many tips and variations to create a wide-ranging gluten-free repertoire.

A modern gluten-free diet is a simple way to get back to feeling fit and healthy. In these pages you'll find delicious, approachable and easy recipes packed with vibrant flavours that you will be happy to share with friends and family. Your guests won't even realize that they are eating gluten-free!

COELIAC DISEASE AND GLUTEN INTOLERANCE

Your diet is a crucial key to good health: it should leave you feeling energized and full of vitality. But for some, what we eat can leave us feeling drained, tired and irritable, with frequent headaches or mouth ulcers, and difficulties with concentration. Gastrointestinal distress can vary from bloating, wind or heartburn to constipation, cramps or diarrhoea, weight gain or weight loss, with similar symptoms to IBS (Irritable Bowel Syndrome), and some people experience joint and muscle pain, and infertility. If your symptoms persist and there is no obvious cause, your doctor can offer you a simple blood test; if positive, he or she will refer you to a consultant for an intestinal biopsy to find out if you have coeliac disease, or severe gluten intolerance.

Coeliac disease is an autoimmune disease in which the body reacts to gluten by producing antibodies – our body's natural defence system – that attack the gluten molecules but also damage the tiny hair-like structures called villi that line the small intestine. These tiny structures help the body absorb essential nutrients from food during digestion, but when damaged and inflamed they cannot work properly, so that many of the nutrients simply pass right through the digestive system, leaving you poorly nourished. The good news is that this damage is not permanent: once you have stopped eating foods that contain gluten, the villi will gradually recover and your body will be able to absorb vital vitamins, minerals, proteins and energy-boosting carbohydrates.

When the villi are damaged, you may also become lactose intolerant or find it difficult to digest milk, yogurt and cheese products. This is because the villi tips produce the enzyme lactase, which is needed to break down and digest the milk sugar lactose. Once the villi are healed you're usually able to tolerate dairy foods.

You may not test positive for coeliac disease but find your symptoms clear up when you eliminate gluten from your diet – this is described as gluten intolerance, and the effects in the intestine are very similar. However, it is a good idea to get retested a year after your initial test, as results can be inconclusive. Even if your

COELIAC DISEASE AND GLUTEN INTOLERANCE
...CONTINUED

symptoms are mild, and you decide to carry on eating gluten, if your intestines are not functioning correctly you risk suffering from vitamin and mineral deficiences, and in the long term this can result in anaemia or osteoporosis.

Changing your diet can have a huge impact on your life, improving your health and well-being and boosting your energy levels.

Wheat allergies
Wheat allergy is different from gluten intolerance. Although both are a result of the body's immune system reacting to food, an allergic response is noticeable soon after eating the food: symptoms vary from a mild rash or sneezing to vomiting, diarrhoea or acute respiratory problems. A food allergy can be diagnosed by a medically supervised skin prick test. With a wheat allergy you can still eat rye and barley – good news for beer drinkers – but a gluten-free diet will help you to avoid trigger foods that contain wheat.

Getting tested
It is important that you do not change your diet or attempt to give up gluten before getting tested by your doctor, otherwise the diagnosis may be inconclusive.

GLUTEN-FREE INGREDIENTS

Gluten is a name for several different proteins (prolamins) found in wheat, rye and barley. If you have recently been diagnosed with coeliac disease, the thought of never being able to eat a slice of your favourite cake or pizza again may leave you feeling a little down. But recent years have seen an explosion of gluten-free products: breads, crackers, luxurious cakes and cookies, pasta, pies, pizza bases, even gluten-free beer – and some of these are available on prescription in the UK.

While you will not be able to cook with wheat flour, a wide range of grains and flours are gluten-free. Some ingredients will be new to you, but you will be familiar with others, such as cornflour and Italian polenta – both of which are made from maize (corn). Gram (chickpea) flour is used widely in Indian cookery. Buckwheat flour is not derived from a cereal grain, but is ground from the small triangular seeds of a plant related to rhubarb; it is known as *sarrasin* in France, where it is used to make crêpes, and as *kasha* in Russia and Poland. Other alternative grains include millet and sorghum, both of which have been grown for thousands of years in India and Africa, and quinoa, a nutritious plant from South America.

Gluten-free flours work best when blended together rather than used on their own. Rice flour (white or brown) or polenta, a pale yellow flour, can be mixed with tapioca flour, milled from the root of the West Indian cassava plant, to make light, fluffy cakes. Rice flour mixed with stronger-tasting buckwheat, quinoa or chestnut flour is great in savoury dishes. Ready-mixed gluten-free plain, self-raising and bread flour blends allow you to make cakes, cookies, breads and pizzas. Ground nuts and seeds, such as flax and sunflower, can also be used to replace some of the flour in cakes, pastries and coatings.

GLUTEN-FREE INGREDIENTS ...CONTINUED

WHAT ABOUT OATS?

Oats contain proteins called avenins; some people with coeliac disease are sensitive to these, but it is now thought they can be tolerated by many. Only introduce oats into your diet under medical supervision or with the approval of your doctor or health consultant Be aware that oats may become contaminated with gluten-containing cereals during harvesting, milling or transportation. Read labels and check oats are gluten-free.

Xanthan gum and guar guar gum

Gluten gives bread its elasticity, enabling it to rise and hold the stretch during baking, and helps pastry to hold together as you roll and shape it. When cooking gluten-free breads and pastries, some recipes call for a small amount of xanthan gum to hold food particles together. Xanthan gum is a corn-based ingredient in the form of a white powder, sold in supermarkets and health food shops. It is stirred into dry ingredients before the addition of eggs, water or milk; be sure to mix the dry ingredients well, or the xanthan gum can taste bitter. Guar gum, made from a type of bean, is used in a similar way. Some cooks prefer it as it is less highly processed than xanthan gum; the downside is that it can have laxative and flatulent effects.

GLUTEN-FREE FOODS

Lots of foods naturally contain no gluten, including:

- Eggs
- Dairy foods – milk, cream, full-fat crème fraîche, plain yogurt (check labels of flavoured yogurts), buttermilk, cheese (some reduced fat soft cheeses and reduced fat crème fraiche or processed cheeses may not be gluten-free)
- Butter, lard (shortening), ghee, margarine, low-fat spreads (some low-fat spreads and margarines may have gluten-containing soy or wheat lecithin added to stop them from separating).
- Fresh, frozen and dried fruit and veg; canned fruit in fruit juice and vegetables in water
- Fresh or frozen meat and poultry, smoked meat
- Fresh, frozen and smoked fish and shellfish; canned fish in brine, oil or springwater
- Plain tofu

GLUTEN-FREE FLOURS

- Arrowroot
- Buckwheat flour
- Carob flour
- Cornflour (cornstarch)
- Fine or medium polenta (cornmeal)
- Gram (chickpea) flour
- Millet flour
- Potato flour, potato starch
- Quinoa flour
- Rice flour
- Sago
- Sorghum flour
- Soya flour
- Tapioca flour
- Teff

GLUTEN-FREE STORECUPBOARD FOODS

- Rice and rice noodles (unflavoured)
- Dried and canned pulses – beans, peas, lentils (check labels of pulses in sauce)
- Nuts and seeds (except dry-roasted and flavoured)
- Oils and vinegars
- Garlic purée, tomato purée (tomato paste)
- Dried herbs
- Freshly ground spices
- Vanilla extract and essence
- Bicarbonate of soda, cream of tartar
- Fresh and dried yeast, yeast extract
- Gelatine
- Sugar, honey, golden syrup and/or corn syrup, treacle, maple syrup
- Jams and jellies
- Wine – red, white, sparkling, sherry, port, vermouth
- Cider
- Spirits and liqueurs

FOODS THAT CAN TRIP YOU UP

A number of foods contain hidden gluten or wheat or barley derivatives. Some products may contain gluten, depending on the manufacturer, so always check the label before buying. Coeliac UK (www.coeliac.org.uk) and, in the US, Celiac Society (www.celiacsociety.com) have a lot of information online and publish directories based on the latest information from manufacturers. Here are some key foods that you may not realise contain gluten:

- Baked beans (most brands contain gluten)
- Baking powder (some brands contain gluten)
- Barley water (plain or flavoured) and pearl barley
- Beers, lager, stouts and ales contain barley malt (look out for gluten-free versions)
- Breakfast cereals sweetened with barley malt extract are not gluten-free; oats cannot be tolerated by some people and may not be guaranteed to be gluten-free
- Bulgur, couscous, semolina, wheat protein, bran, rusk, starch and wheat germ are all different ways to process wheat grain
- Chocolate is naturally gluten-free, but cross-contamination may occur during processing
- Chutneys (some brands contain wheat flour)
- Coffee from vending machines
- Corn tortillas
- Curry powder (some brands may contain gluten)
- Dry-roasted nuts and Bombay mix
- Durum, einkorn, emmer, kamut and spelt are all varieties of wheat. Triticale is a hybrid grain from wheat and rye
- Flavoured crisps (some types contain gluten); the plain or lightly salted flavours are usually gluten-free
- Malted milk drinks
- Marzipan and ready-made icing (some brands may include wheat products)
- Mustard: pure mustard powder is usually gluten-free, but some readymade mustards and mustard sauces include wheat flour
- Pâté and breaded ham
- Peanut butter: nuts are gluten-free, but some nut butters may be cross-contaminated during manufacturing
- Potato products such as oven chips may be coated in wheat flour to keep the chips separate
- Ready-made salad dressings and sauces
- Sausages, burgers and Scotch eggs may contain wheat rusk
- Soy sauce, teriyaki and tamari sauce generally contain wheat or barley, although gluten-free versions are available
- Stock cubes, gravy granules and seasoning mixes; look carefully at dried soup and noodle mixes too
- Stuffing mixes and breadcrumb coatings on fishfingers, fish fillets and chicken
- Suet: shredded suet is coated in wheat flour to keep it free-flowing, although gluten-free versions are available
- Tomato ketchup
- White pepper may be ground and bulked with wheat flour

FOODS THAT CONTAIN GLUTEN

Common foods that contain gluten include:

- Bread (white and wholemeal), pitta and naan breads, crumpets, bagels and muffins
- Biscuits (cookies) and cakes
- Crackers and crispbreads
- Pasta and noodles
- Pizza
- Pastries, pies, tarts and sausage rolls
- Battered fish and tempura
- Pancakes, crêpes and blini

LEARN TO LOVE THOSE LABELS

Packaged foods sometimes contain unexpected ingredients, so always read the labels and check the ingredients list before you buy. The manufacturer must list wheat, rye, barley, oats, spelt and kamut if they are included. Look for the crossed grain symbol to show that the item is gluten-free, or for allergy advice; however, this is not compulsory, so not all manufacturers include it on their labels.

More and more supermarkets stock a range of 'free from' foods to make sourcing gluten-free basics quick and easy while doing the family shopping. Check gluten-free specialist directories or online so that you are aware of new ingredients. If you are unsure then don't be afraid to telephone a manufacturer directly to make certain that the ingredient really is gluten-free.

A food that is labelled wheat free is not automatically gluten-free, as it may contain barley or rye.

GOOD KITCHEN PRACTICE

Gluten molecules are invisible to the naked eye, and it is all-too-easy to cross-contaminate gluten-free foods with tiny particles of a gluten-containing ingredients. Anyone sharing a kitchen with someone who is gluten intolerant needs to be vigilant in order to avoid cross-contamination.

- Ideally, use separate chopping boards, knives, sieves, colanders, rolling pins and other basic equipment. Mark them clearly and keep in a separate 'gluten-free' cupboard.
- Always wipe kitchen surfaces with a clean cloth before you begin cooking.
- When measuring butter, always use a clean knife.
- Use clean oil when frying to avoid cross-contamination from gluten-containing ingredients.
- Breakfast toast can be tricky, especially if everyone's in a rush. A butter knife used to spread butter on wheat toast can leave crumbs in the butter dish.

Keep a separate butter dish, clearly marked for gluten-intolerant family members. Use toaster bags for gluten-free bread, or use the toaster only for wheat bread and a clean grill for gluten-free toast.

- Use a teaspoon to spoon out jam, rather than a knife that may have been used on wheat toast. Squeezy bottles of honey, mayo and gluten-free ketchup can also help prevent contamination.

Make two, freeze on
Make a double-sized supper at the weekend, enjoy half and freeze the remainder in wrapped single portions for nights when you are too tired to cook. Or look for this ⊙ symbol to indicate dishes that can be served cold the next day.

Love your freezer
Guten-free bread stales quickly, so keep a supply of sliced bread in the freezer and take out only as much as you need. Same goes for cakes and puddings: wrap, label and freeze as single portions.

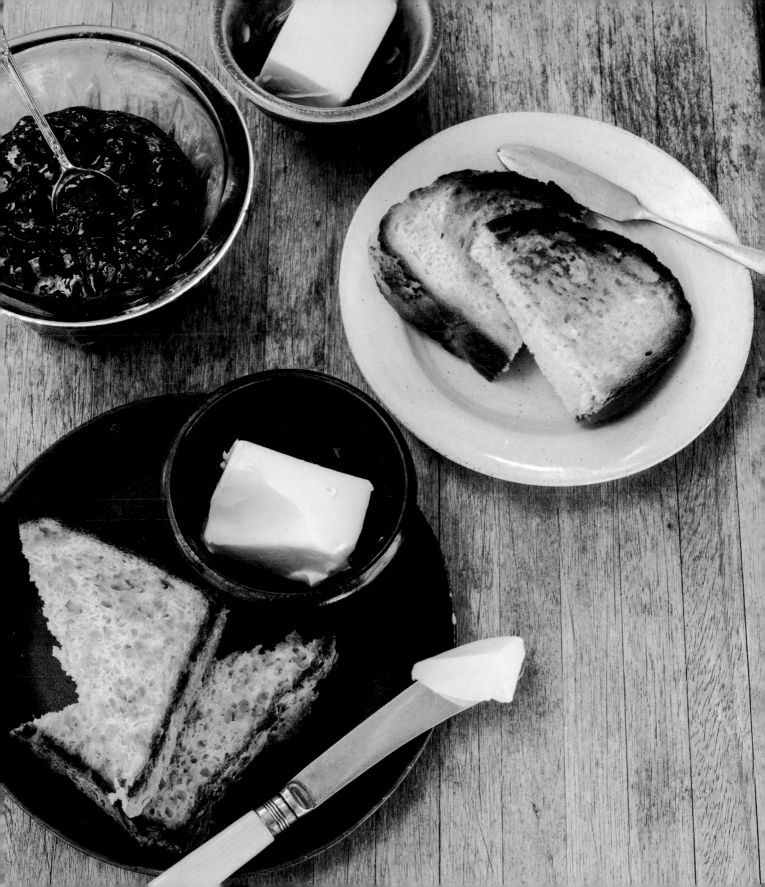

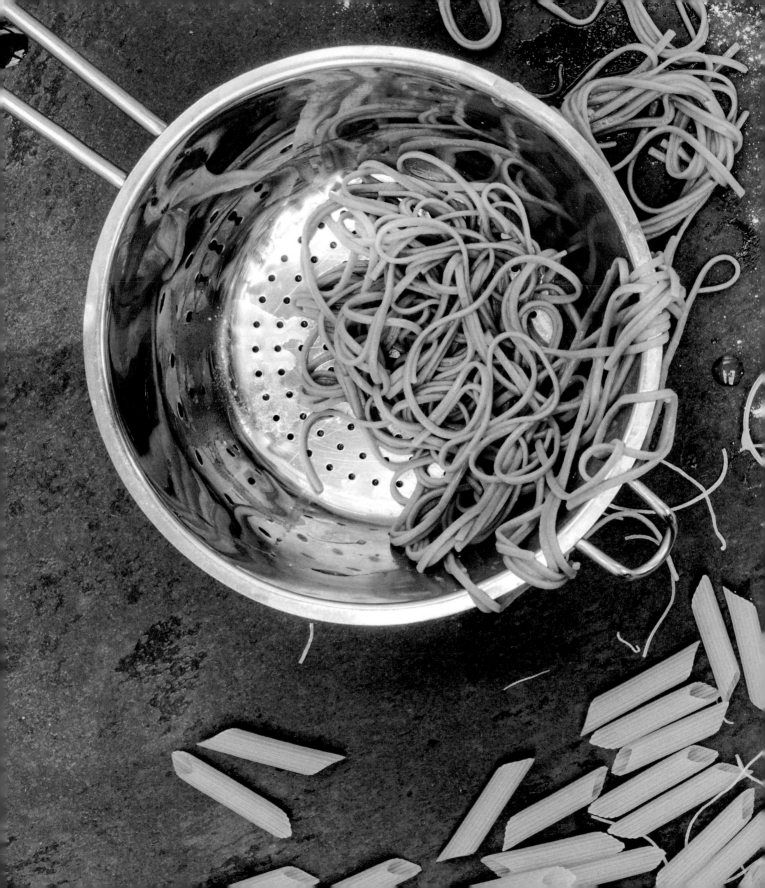

PASTA, GNOCCHI & NOODLES

PASTA, GNOCCHI & NOODLES

In recent years the availability of gluten-free foods has steadily increased in all the main supermarket chains. For example, you can now buy dried corn pasta in various shapes. It makes a speedy basis for a midweek supper and cooks in just the same way as its wheat-based counterpart.

Italian gnocchi (little dumplings) are not gluten free if bought ready-made, but they are easy to make at home by replacing the wheat flour with a gluten-free flour; flavour them with fresh herbs or rocket (arugula).

Toss pasta or gnocchi with a simple tomato sauce made with garlicky fried onions simmered with chopped tomatoes and flavoured with fresh herbs. Pesto-style sauces are naturally gluten free and quick to make: blitz fresh basil with olive oil and pine nuts or ground almonds. Rocket or spinach leaves, walnuts, olives and sun-dried tomatoes also work well in pesto.

For a gluten-free cheese sauce, mix a tablespoonful or two of cornflour (cornstarch) or arrowroot with a little milk to make a paste, add a knob of butter and plenty more milk to make a sauce and bring to the boil, whisking until thickened and smooth. Flavour with grated cheese and mustard. Always check the labels: although cornflour (cornstarch) and mustard are naturally gluten free they are sometimes sold mixed with wheat flour.

In Asian-inspired recipes choose rice noodles: they are naturally gluten free and are available in a range of sizes, from thick ribbons to fine, hair-like strands. Japanese soba noodles are made with buckwheat (which is gluten free) and make a great base for clear soups or stews; check the labels, and choose the type that's 100 per cent buckwheat (and wheat free).

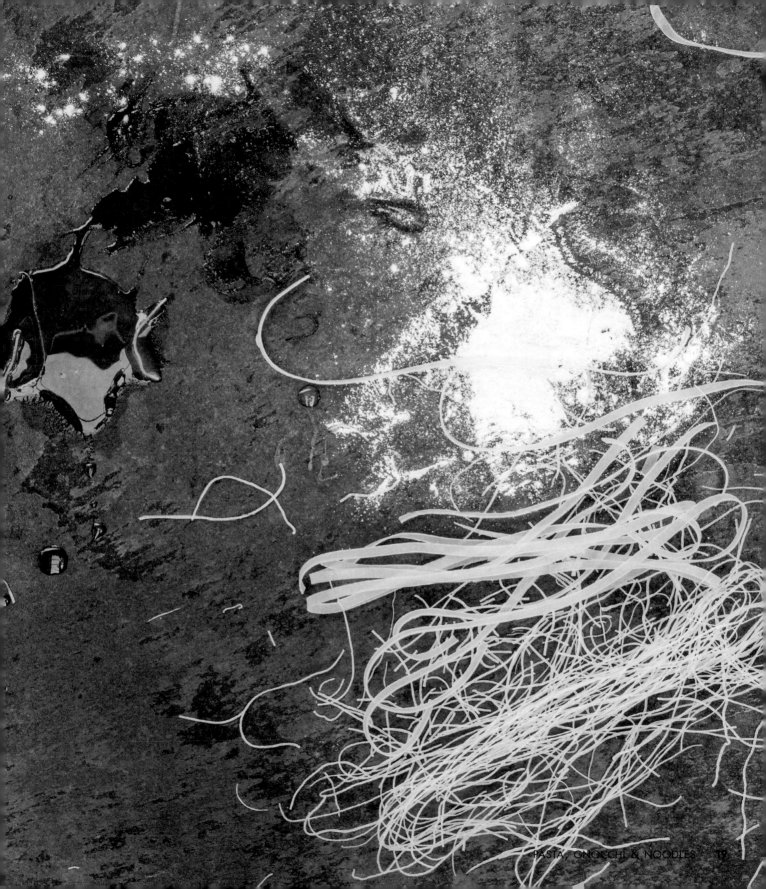

GAME LASAGNE
WITH SAGE BÉCHAMEL

SERVES 4

PREP: 50 MINUTES, PLUS 30 MINUTES STANDING TIME

COOK: 2 HOURS

250g/9oz GLUTEN-FREE DRIED LASAGNE SHEETS
4 TBSP FRESHLY GRATED PARMESAN CHEESE

Game casserole

1 TBSP OLIVE OIL
750g/1lb 10oz BONELESS DICED VENISON OR A MIX OF
    DICED VENISON, PHEASANT AND PIGEON
1 RED ONION, CHOPPED
200g/7oz CHESTNUT (CREMINI) MUSHROOMS,
    QUARTERED
2 GARLIC CLOVES, FINELY CHOPPED
1 TBSP RICE FLOUR
200ml/7fl oz/GENEROUS ¾ CUP RED WINE
450ml/16fl oz/2 CUPS GLUTEN-FREE BEEF STOCK
1 TBSP TOMATO PURÉE (TOMATO PASTE)
1 TBSP REDCURRANT JELLY
½ TSP JUNIPER BERRIES, ROUGHLY CRUSHED
SALT AND FRESHLY GROUND BLACK PEPPER

Sage béchamel

600ml/20fl oz/2½ CUPS MILK
3 SPRIGS OF FRESH SAGE, LEAVES ONLY
½ ONION, THINLY SLICED
3 TBSP GLUTEN-FREE CORNFLOUR (CORNSTARCH)
25g/1oz/2 TBSP UNSALTED BUTTER

Lasagne is one of those trusted suppers that can be prepped earlier in the day and kept in the fridge ready to bake later. This luxury version is made with diced venison or mixed game (available in larger supermarkets); alternatively, use the same amount of lean diced lamb or braising beef instead.

1. Preheat the oven to 160°C/325°F/Gas Mark 3. Heat the oil in a large frying pan, add the game a few pieces at a time until it has all been added, then cook over a high heat, stirring until browned. Using a slotted spoon, transfer to a casserole dish.

2. Add the onion to the pan and cook for about 5 minutes over a medium heat, until softened. Add the mushrooms and garlic and cook for 2–3 minutes, until the mushrooms begin to colour. Stir in the flour, then mix in the wine, stock, tomato purée, redcurrant jelly and juniper. Season generously with salt and pepper and bring to the boil. Pour over the game, cover and cook in the oven for 1¼ hours, or until tender. Leave to cool.

3. To make the béchamel, pour the milk into a saucepan, add the sage leaves, onion, salt and pepper. Bring to the boil, then remove from the heat, cover and leave to stand for 30 minutes.

4. Strain the milk into a bowl, reserving the sage leaves. Add the cornflour to the milk pan and gradually whisk in the strained milk, until smooth. Add the butter and bring to the boil, whisking until thickened and smooth.

5. Spoon half the game casserole into a 2.5 litre/4½ pint/2½ quart square dish. Cover with one-third of the lasagne sheets. Pour over just under half the béchamel, then cover with half the remaining lasagne sheets, then the remaining game. Cover with the last of the lasagne sheets and the béchamel. Press a few of the reserved sage leaves on top, then sprinkle with the Parmesan.

6. Bake for 40–45 minutes, until the top is golden brown, the sauces are bubbling and the pasta is tender. Serve with salad.

Cook's tip There is no need to cook the lasagne sheets first, but make sure you press them down into the sauces, especially the top layer, or the sheets may curl up as they cook. If they do, simply press back down with a spoon and continue cooking.

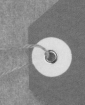

Freezing tip The cooked game casserole can be frozen in a plastic bag for up to 3 months. Thaw overnight in the fridge. Make the sauce and add the lasagne sheets up to 4 hours before serving (keep in the fridge until ready to bake).

VIETNAMESE NOODLE SALAD

SERVES 4

PREP: 20 MINUTES

COOK: 5 MINUTES

🍽️⊙🍴

200g/7oz DRIED THIN RICE NOODLES

2 TBSP SESAME SEEDS

2 TBSP SUNFLOWER SEEDS

2 TBSP GLUTEN-FREE TAMARI SAUCE

GRATED ZEST AND JUICE OF 2 LIMES

4 TBSP SUNFLOWER OIL

FRESHLY GROUND BLACK PEPPER

Salad

1 LARGE CARROT, CUT INTO THIN MATCHSTICKS

¼ CUCUMBER, HALVED, DESEEDED AND
    CUT INTO THIN MATCHSTICKS

2 SPRING ONIONS (SCALLIONS),
    CUT INTO THIN MATCHSTICKS

115g/4oz BEAN SPROUTS, RINSED AND DRAINED

175g/6oz CHINESE LEAVES (CHINESE CABBAGE),
    THINLY SHREDDED

SMALL BUNCH OF FRESH MINT, FINELY CHOPPED

175g/6oz COLD COOKED CHICKEN,
    SHREDDED INTO SMALL PIECES

Cook's tip Salad dressings can make a leafy salad go limp if added in advance. To get round this for a lunchbox, dress the noodles, top with the chicken or other flavouring, then spoon the salad on top. Stir together just before serving.

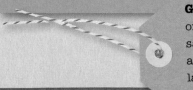

GF tip Soy sauce and some brands of tamari (a thicker, Japanese soy sauce) contain wheat or barley and are not gluten-free: check the labels carefully.

Chinese rice noodles make a great base for a main-course salad and any leftovers can be packed into a plastic box for lunch the next day. A good way to stretch leftover roast chicken.

1. Cook the noodles in boiling water for 2 minutes or as pack directs, until just tender. Drain and rinse in cold water. Heat a small frying pan over a medium–high heat and dry-fry the sesame and sunflower seeds, shaking the pan until evenly browned. Remove from the heat, add the tamari and leave to cool.

2. Mix the lime zest and juice with the oil, seeds and tamari, and a little pepper, then toss with the cooled noodles. Spoon into a salad bowl or 4 individual plastic lunchboxes.

3. To make the salad, toss together all the salad ingredients except the chicken. Scatter the chicken over the noodles, then top with the salad. If taking to work or school the next day, cover and chill. If serving now, toss the salad together, then spoon into bowls.

OTHER FLAVOUR COMBOS

Instead of cold cooked chicken, try:
- 2 x 150g/5½oz salmon steaks, steamed, microwaved or grilled, then flaked into pieces.
- 200g/7oz canned tuna in spring water, drained and flaked.
- 200g/7oz frozen prawns (shrimp), thawed, rinsed with cold water and drained well.
- 200g/7oz firm tofu, sliced and drizzled with a little gluten-free tamari sauce, sesame oil and some chopped fresh ginger, then grilled and cooled.
- 3 eggs beaten with 1 tbsp water and some dried red chilli flakes, cooked in a frying pan with a little sunflower oil to make a thin omelette. Cool and cut into thin shreds.

Or try:
- Little Gem or iceberg lettuce instead of Chinese leaves.
- Fresh coriander (cilantro) or basil instead of mint.

PAD THAI

SERVES 4
PREP: 10 MINUTES, PLUS 6–8 MINUTES SOAKING
COOK: 10 MINUTES

250g/9oz DRIED FLAT RICE NOODLES
2 TBSP SUNFLOWER OIL
2 CARROTS, CUT INTO MATCHSTICKS
4 SPRING ONIONS (SCALLIONS),
    CUT INTO MATCHSTICKS
2 GARLIC CLOVES, FINELY CHOPPED
225g/8oz FROZEN KING PRAWNS (SHRIMP),
    THAWED, RINSED AND DRAINED
300g/10½oz BEAN SPROUTS,
    RINSED AND DRAINED
2 EGGS
2–3 TBSP GLUTEN-FREE THAI FISH SAUCE
2 TSP LIGHT MUSCOVADO (BROWN) SUGAR
1 LARGE MILD FRESH RED CHILLI,
    DESEEDED AND FINELY CHOPPED
JUICE OF 1 LIME
40g/1½oz SALTED PEANUTS, ROUGHLY CHOPPED
LARGE HANDFUL OF FRESH CORIANDER (CILANTRO) LEAVES,
    ROUGHLY CHOPPED

To garnish

¼ CUCUMBER, CUT INTO THIN STRIPS
2 TBSP SALTED PEANUTS, CHOPPED
LIME WEDGES

Need supper in a hurry? Here is the answer. Thaw the prawns in a bowl of cold water as soon as you get home, change the water several times and they will be ready to use in 30 minutes or so.

1. Cook the noodles in boiling water for 5 minutes or as pack directs, until just tender.

2. Heat the oil in a wok, add the carrots and stir-fry for 2 minutes. Add the spring onions and garlic and stir-fry for 1 minute. Add the prawns and stir-fry for 2 minutes. Tip in the bean sprouts and stir-fry for 1–2 minutes, until hot.

3. Beat the eggs with 2 tbsp fish sauce, the sugar, chilli and lime juice. Drain the noodles, add to the wok together with the peanuts and egg mixture and stir-fry until the egg is just beginning to cook and the prawns are piping hot. Taste and add more fish sauce if needed.

4. Sprinkle in the coriander. Spoon into bowls and garnish with the cucumber and a few peanuts. Serve with lime wedges and squeeze over some lime juice to taste.

Cook's tip This is a great recipe to adapt depending on what you have in the fridge: you could add some leftover cooked chicken or roast pork, shredded into small pieces; diced tofu and mushrooms; or a few mangetout (snow peas), leeks or green beans.

GF tip If flat rice noodles are not available in your local supermarket, look for them in Asian food shops.

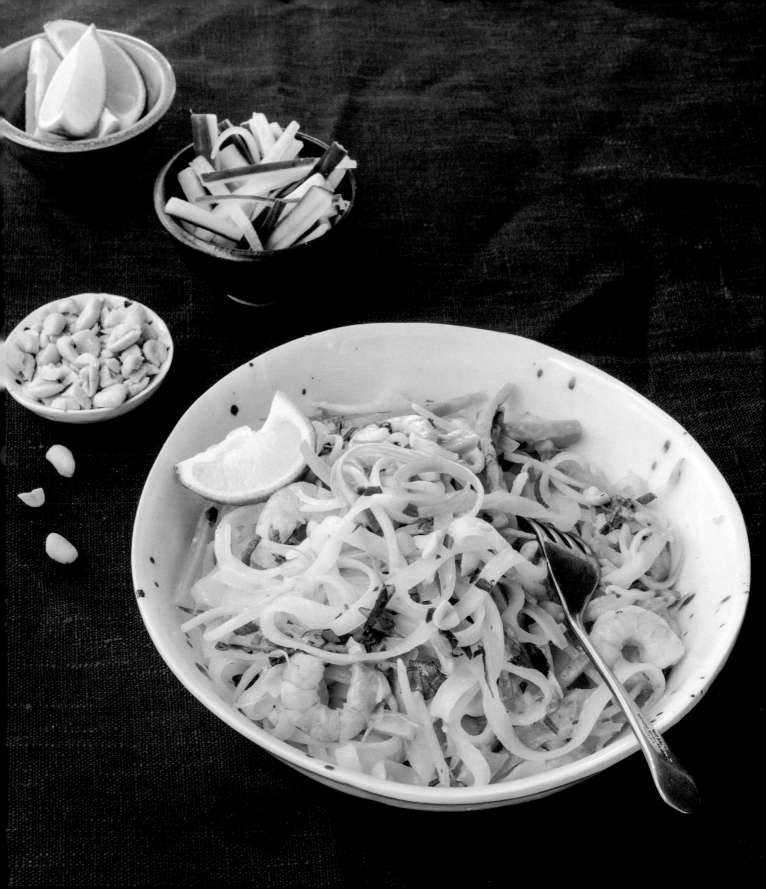

PEA AND ROCKET
GNOCCHI
WITH FRESH PESTO

SERVES 4

PREP: 25 MINUTES

COOK: 25 MINUTES

650g/1lb 7oz POTATOES, PEELED AND CUT INTO CHUNKS
200g/7oz/1½ CUPS FROZEN PEAS
115g/4oz/½ CUP RICOTTA CHEESE
55g/2oz PARMESAN CHEESE, GRATED
3 EGG YOLKS
55g/2oz/½ CUP QUINOA FLOUR
1 TSP GLUTEN-FREE BAKING POWDER
PINCH OF GRATED NUTMEG
SALT AND FRESHLY GROUND BLACK PEPPER
70g/2½oz ROCKET (ARUGULA) LEAVES

Pesto

55g/2oz PARMESAN CHEESE, GRATED,
   PLUS EXTRA TO GARNISH
55g/2oz/7 TBSP PINE NUTS
25g/1oz FRESH BASIL LEAVES,
   PLUS EXTRA TO GARNISH
250ml/9fl oz/1 CUP EXTRA VIRGIN OLIVE OIL

These mini potato and pea dumplings make a light, summery supper. Don't be tempted to use leftover cooked potato, as this will make heavy dumplings.

1. To make the gnocchi, add the potatoes to a saucepan of boiling water and simmer for 15 minutes, until just tender.

2. Meanwhile, make the pesto: put the Parmesan, pine nuts and basil in a blender and blend until finely chopped. With the motor running, gradually trickle in the oil until it has all been added; transfer to a small bowl and set aside.

3. Add the peas to the potatoes and cook for 3 minutes, then drain into a colander and return to the pan. Mash the potatoes and peas, then add the ricotta, Parmesan and egg yolks and mash together until well mixed. Stir in the flour and baking powder. Season generously with nutmeg, salt and pepper. Chop half the rocket leaves and stir into the potato mixture.

4. Roll the mixture into long sausage shapes, about 2.5cm/1in thick, then chill for 15 minutes. Cut diagonally into short pieces and flatten each piece slightly with the prongs of a fork.

5. Bring a large saucepan of water to the boil, drop in half the gnocchi piece by piece and simmer for 3–4 minutes, or until the little dumplings rise to the surface of the water. Scoop out onto a plate with a slotted spoon, and keep hot while you cook the remaining gnocchi.

6. Serve the gnocchi in shallow bowls, drizzle the pesto over, and garnish with the remaining rocket, a few basil leaves and a little grated Parmesan.

Recipe continues...

GF tip Quinoa flour adds a slightly nutty taste to these dumplings; if you don't have any, substitute brown rice flour.

Cook's tip Gnocchi can also be shaped using 2 teaspoons: scoop a little of the mixture onto a spoon, then scoop onto a second spoon to even up the shape, then scoop onto a chopping board to form a neat quenelle or small oval shape – it sounds much more complicated than it actually is and once you have had a go, it is easy to speed up. Flatten slightly with a fork for the characteristic pattern, which holds the sauce.

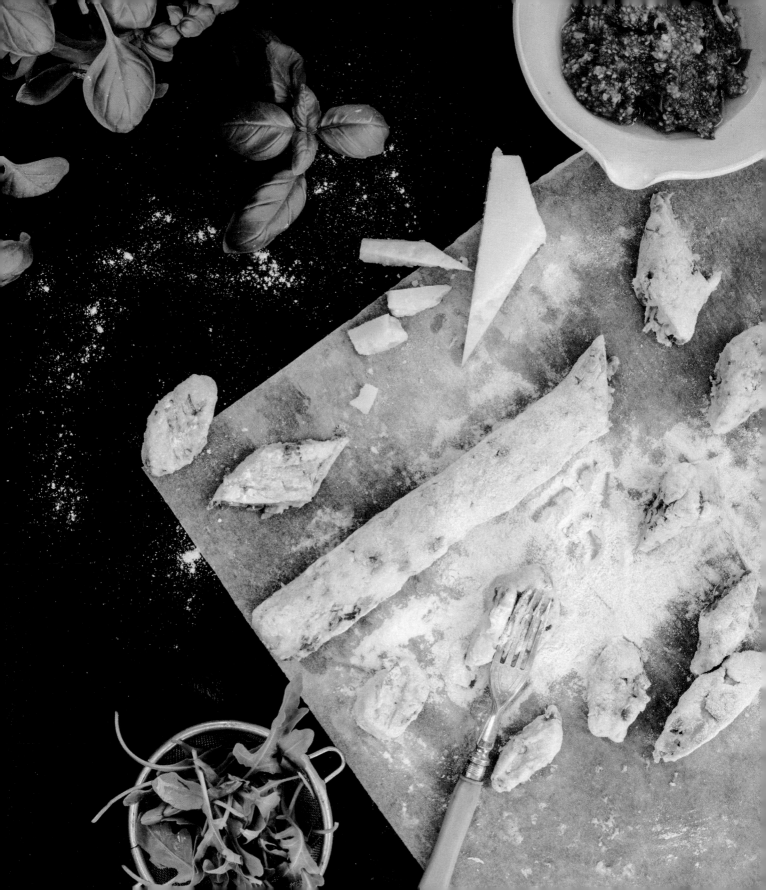

SUN-DRIED TOMATO GNOCCHI WITH PUTTANESCA SAUCE

Omit the peas and rocket from the gnocchi. When mashing the potatoes add 85g/3oz drained and chopped sun-dried tomatoes in oil. Shape as in step 4. Instead of the pesto, make a sauce by frying 1 chopped onion in 1 tbsp olive oil until softened. Add 2 chopped garlic cloves and a 400g can of chopped tomatoes, flavour with a small handful of basil leaves, 55g/2oz stoned and chopped black olives, 1 tsp caster (superfine) sugar, salt and pepper. Simmer for 5 minutes, until thick, stirring from time to time. Cook the gnocchi as in step 5. Spoon into bowls, spoon over the tomato sauce and garnish with extra basil leaves.

PASTITSIO

SERVES 4
PREP: 30 MINUTES
COOK: 1¼ HOURS

1 TBSP OLIVE OIL
500g/1lb 2oz MINCED (GROUND) LAMB
1 ONION, FINELY CHOPPED
2 GARLIC CLOVES, FINELY CHOPPED
1 AUBERGINE (EGGPLANT), DICED
1 RED PEPPER, CORED, DESEEDED AND DICED
400g CAN CHOPPED TOMATOES
200ml/7fl oz/GENEROUS ¾ CUP GLUTEN-FREE
    LAMB STOCK
200ml/7fl oz/GENEROUS ¾ CUP RED WINE
    OR EXTRA STOCK
1 TBSP TOMATO PURÉE (TOMATO PASTE)
2 SPRIGS OF FRESH ROSEMARY
½ TSP GROUND CINNAMON
PINCH OF GRATED NUTMEG, PLUS EXTRA FOR THE TOPPING
SALT AND FRESHLY GROUND BLACK PEPPER

Topping

350g/12oz GLUTEN-FREE DRIED PENNE PASTA
300g/10½oz/1¼ CUPS GLUTEN-FREE REDUCED-FAT
    CREAM CHEESE
2 EGGS
2 SPRIGS OF FRESH ROSEMARY, LEAVES FINELY CHOPPED
85g/3oz PARMESAN CHEESE, GRATED

Everyone loves spaghetti Bolognese, and this Greek-style oven-baked pasta dish is a delicious variation on the theme. Cook the meat base up to a day ahead (or freeze it), then finish off with the pasta topping and bake when needed. Serve with a crisp green salad.

1. Heat the oil in a saucepan, add the lamb and onion and fry for 5 minutes, breaking up the meat with a spoon and stirring until the meat is evenly browned. Mix in the garlic, aubergine and red pepper and cook for 3–4 minutes.

2. Mix in the tomatoes, lamb stock and red wine, then the tomato purée, rosemary, spices, salt and pepper. Bring to the boil, cover and simmer for 45 minutes, stirring from time to time.

3. When the meat is almost ready, preheat the oven to 190°C/ 375°F/Gas Mark 5. Add the pasta to a large saucepan of boiling water and cook until al dente. Drain in a colander.

4. Add the cream cheese to the pasta pan, whisk in the eggs, then the chopped rosemary, a little nutmeg and plenty of salt and pepper. Gently stir in the pasta to coat evenly.

5. Spoon the meat mixture into a 2.5 litre/4½ pint/2½ quart ovenproof dish, discarding the rosemary sprigs. Spoon the pasta mixture in an even layer over the top. Sprinkle with the Parmesan and bake for 30–35 minutes, until the topping is golden. Serve immediately, with a green salad.

GF tip Instead of a flour-based sauce, reduced-fat cream cheese makes a speedy sauce when tossed with freshly cooked gluten-free pasta and warmed through. Add chopped herbs, garlic or other flavourings. Great with diced cooked chicken and bacon, mushrooms, or salmon. If the sauce is very thick, add a splash of stock or milk, white wine or lemon juice.

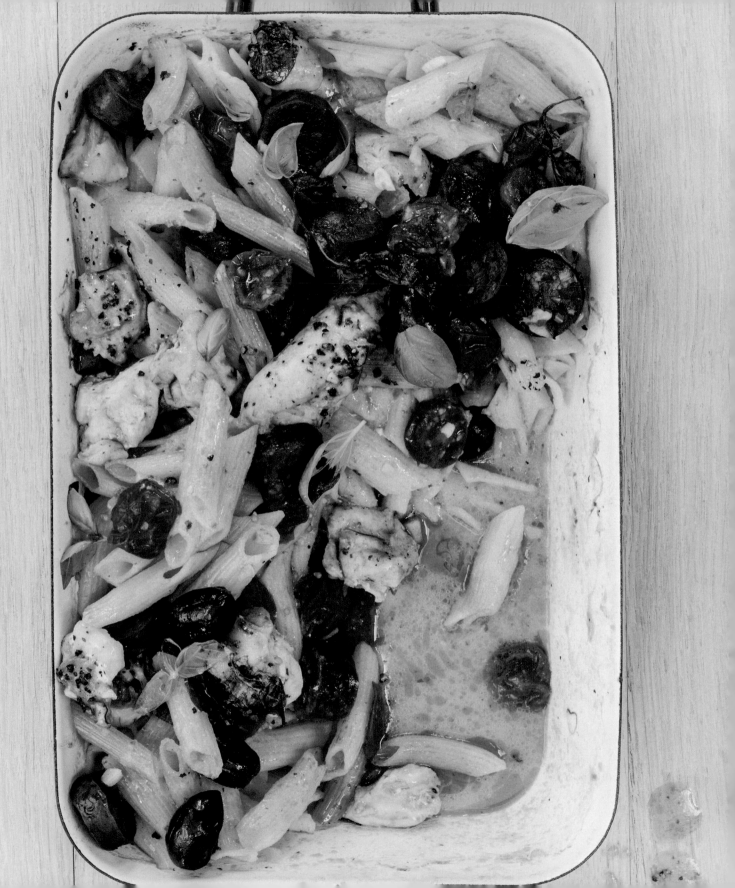

CHICKEN AND CHORIZO
PASTA BAKE

SERVES 4–6

PREP: 20 MINUTES

COOK: 1 HOUR

1.2 LITRES/2 PINTS/5 CUPS GLUTEN-FREE CHICKEN STOCK

LARGE PINCH OF SAFFRON THREADS

500g/1lb 2oz GLUTEN-FREE DRIED PENNE PASTA

3 GARLIC CLOVES, FINELY CHOPPED

HANDFUL OF BASIL LEAVES, PLUS EXTRA TO GARNISH

SALT AND FRESHLY GROUND BLACK PEPPER

250g/9oz CHERRY TOMATOES, HALVED

450g/1lb BONELESS, SKINLESS CHICKEN THIGHS,
    EACH CUT INTO 4 OR 5 CHUNKS

250g/9oz GLUTEN-FREE CHORIZO SAUSAGE,
    THICKLY SLICED

70g/2½oz MARINATED BLACK OLIVES

2 TBSP OLIVE OIL

Saffron adds the most wonderful flavour and colour to a simple chicken dish. As everything is baked in one dish, this makes a perfect Friday night supper to share with friends or family, leaving you time to relax while it cooks.

1. Preheat the oven to 180°C/350°F/Gas Mark 4. Bring the stock to the boil in a saucepan, stir in the saffron and leave to stand for 5 minutes.

2. Put the pasta into a 2.8 litre/5 pint/3 quart casserole dish. Stir the garlic into the hot saffron stock and then pour over the pasta. Tear the basil over the top, season with salt and pepper, then stir to separate the pasta. Scatter the tomato halves, chicken, chorizo and olives on top.

3. Drizzle with the oil, cover and cook for 30 minutes. Remove the cover and stir, then return to the oven, uncovered, for 20–30 minutes, until the chicken is browned and cooked through and the top is golden. Garnish with basil leaves and serve in shallow bowls, accompanied by a green salad.

Cook's tip If you don't have a large dish with a lid, cover with foil or a baking sheet.

GF tip Homemade stock will give the best flavour, but a gluten-free stock cube dissolved in boiling water will work too. Look for cubes labelled 'low salt' or 'reduced salt' to avoid overpowering the delicate flavour of the saffron.

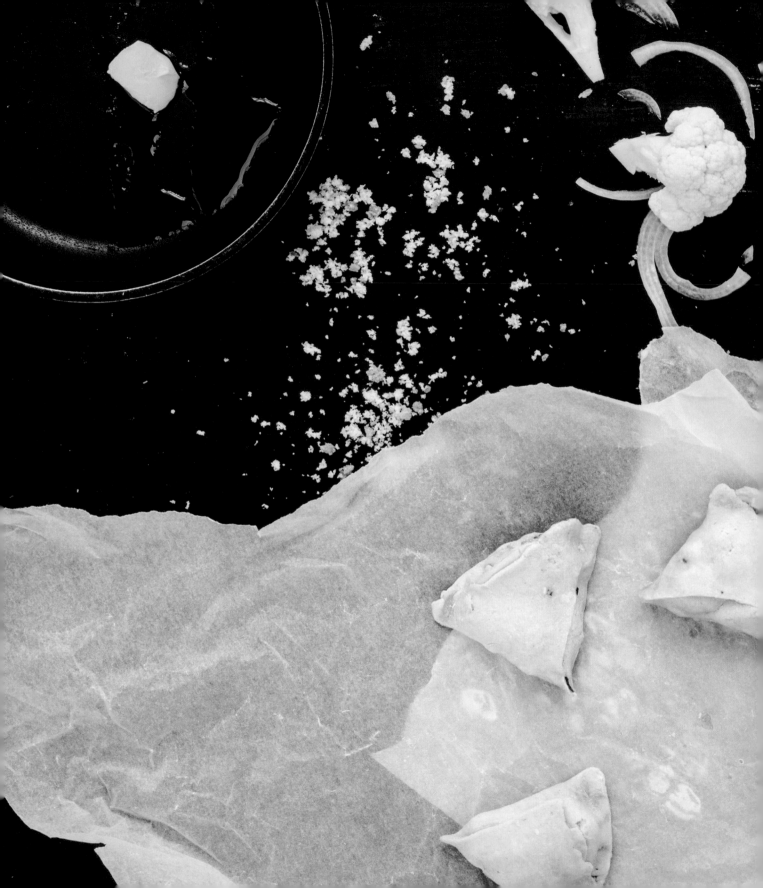

FRIES

FRIES

You can make gluten-free versions of your favourite fries at home. The important thing is to avoid cross-contamination: use fresh oil, or reuse oil that has been used exclusively for gluten-free foods – cool, then strain and label as gluten-free.

Fritto misto is a Mediterranean version of deep-fried fish and shellfish in a light (and, in this case, gluten-free) batter; you can use the same batter for traditional fried fish, or tempura-style veg.

For fans of Indian food there's no need to miss out on onion bhajis (page 41) and samosas (page 42). Make your own bhajis in less time than it would take to wait for a takeaway; samosas can be made in advance and frozen, ready for when you need them.

A gastro-pub favourite, Scotch eggs are easy to adapt to a gluten-free treat (page 34). With a coating of minced pork flavoured with thyme and mustard, and a crisp outer layer of sunflower seeds (or gluten-free breadcrumbs), they're delicious hot or cold.

Keep a supply of breadcrumbs made from a gluten-free loaf in the freezer and use to make your own fish fingers or chicken dippers (or use to coat fish cakes – see page 36). Cut raw fish or chicken breasts into thin strips, coat lightly with rice flour, then dip in beaten egg and finally coat in gluten-free breadcrumbs. Shallow-fry in oil, or spray with a little oil and bake in the oven until crisp and golden.

Crêpes and pancakes need not be made with wheat flour. In France, savoury crêpes are often made with naturally gluten-free buckwheat flour. French-style crêpes or thick American-style pancakes can also be made with a polenta and rice or tapioca flour batter (page 39).

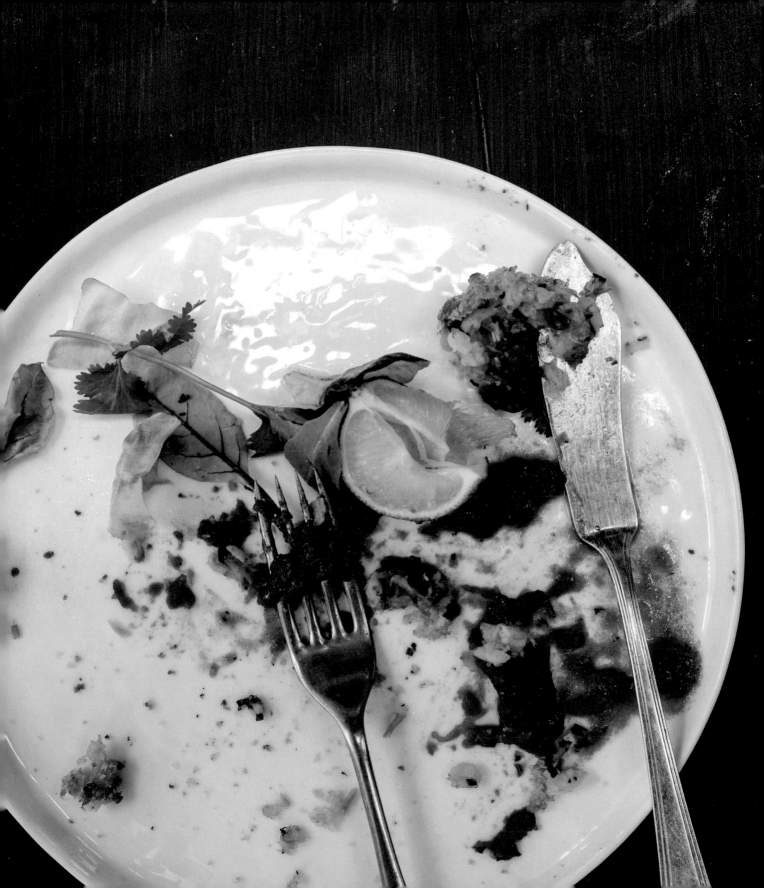

MUSTARD SCOTCH EGGS

MAKES 8
PREP: 50 MINUTES
COOK: 25 MINUTES

🍽️

10 EGGS
3 SPRING ONIONS (SCALLIONS)
2–3 SPRIGS OF THYME, LEAVES ONLY
1½ TSP GLUTEN-FREE MUSTARD POWDER,
    SUCH AS COLMAN'S
1 TSP BLACK PEPPERCORNS, ROUGHLY CRUSHED
¼ TSP SALT
¼ TSP DRIED CHILLI FLAKES (OPTIONAL)
500g/1lb 2oz MINCED (GROUND) PORK
4 TBSP RICE FLOUR, PLUS EXTRA FOR DUSTING
2 TBSP SEMI-SKIMMED (LOW-FAT) MILK
115g/4oz SUNFLOWER SEEDS, FINELY GROUND
1 LITRE/1¾ PINTS/4 CUPS SUNFLOWER OIL
    FOR DEEP-FRYING

Cook's tip Don't be tempted to miss out the chilling stage, or the pork coating may crack when fried.

If you are planning a picnic, these make a pleasant change from sandwiches or a quiche. They're also a great treat for your lunchbox, and they'll keep in the fridge for up to three days. If eight are too many, simply halve the recipe.

1. Put 8 eggs in a saucepan so that they fit quite close together, add cold water to just cover, then bring to the boil over a high heat. Cover and simmer for 6 minutes. Drain, rinse under cold water and crack the shells, then peel as soon as they are cool enough to handle.

2. Finely chop the spring onions in a food processor, add the thyme, mustard powder, pepper, salt and chilli, if using, then the pork. Blitz until the pork is very finely chopped, then mix in 2 tbsp rice flour. Divide into 8 mounds.

3. Roll the eggs in 2 tbsp rice flour, then dust your hands with a little extra flour. Press one of the pork mounds into a thin flat oval shape, either on a chopping board or in the palm of your hand. Add one of the boiled eggs, then wrap the pork mixture around and press the edges together well to completely enclose the egg in a thin, even layer of pork. Set aside on a plate. Continue until all the boiled eggs are coated in the pork. Wrap each one tightly in clingfilm (plastic wrap) and chill for 30 minutes.

4. Beat the 2 remaining eggs with the milk in a shallow dish. Put the ground sunflower seeds on a plate. Roll the pork-covered eggs in a little extra rice flour, then coat in the beaten eggs, then roll in the sunflower seeds.

5. Pour the oil into a deep pan and heat to 180–190°C/350–375°F, or until a cube of bread browns in 30 seconds. Unwrap the eggs, discarding the clingfilm. Using a slotted spoon, lower 2 or 3 eggs carefully into the oil and cook for 4 minutes so that the pork cooks right through, gently turning once or twice so that they brown evenly.

6. Carefully lift out of the oil with a slotted spoon and drain on kitchen paper. Cook the remaining Scotch eggs in the same way, keeping the oil at a constant temperature. Serve warm or cold with salad and gluten-free mustard powder mixed with a little water.

GF tips

Not all mustard is gluten-free, so check the label before using.

Traditionally Scotch eggs are made with sausage meat, but this often contains wheat rusk (they are also rolled in breadcrumbs). Flavoured gluten-free sausages could be used instead of the minced pork; slit and remove the skins and press into oval shapes, as in step 3.

SALMON AND CORIANDER
FISH CAKES

SERVES 4

PREP: 25 MINUTES, PLUS 15–30 MINUTES CHILLING

COOK: 35 MINUTES

500g/1lb 2oz POTATOES, PEELED AND CUT INTO CHUNKS
500g/1lb 2oz SALMON FILLET, CUT INTO 3 PIECES
SALT AND FRESHLY GROUND BLACK PEPPER
25g/1oz/2 TBSP UNSALTED BUTTER
3 SPRING ONIONS (SCALLIONS), FINELY CHOPPED
GRATED ZEST OF 1 LIME
3 TBSP CHOPPED FRESH CORIANDER (CILANTRO) LEAVES
½ –1 LARGE MILD FRESH RED CHILLI,
    DESEEDED AND FINELY CHOPPED
2CM/¾IN PIECE OF FRESH GINGER,
    PEELED AND GRATED
2 TBSP RICE FLOUR
2 EGGS
115g/4oz/GENEROUS 1 CUP DRIED GLUTEN-FREE
    BREADCRUMBS
OLIVE OIL FOR BRUSHING OR SPRAYING
LIME WEDGES, TO SERVE

Quick tomato and coriander chutney

2 TBSP OLIVE OIL
1 GARLIC CLOVE, THINLY SLICED
2CM/¾IN PIECE OF FRESH GINGER,
    PEELED AND GRATED
400g CAN CHOPPED TOMATOES
1 TSP CASTER (SUPERFINE) SUGAR
2 TBSP CHOPPED FRESH CORIANDER (CILANTRO)

Make these Asian-inspired fish cakes earlier in the day (or freeze them); when you're ready to eat, bake in the oven or pan-fry for 8–10 minutes, turning once, until crisp and golden. Delicious with this easy, garlicky tomato chutney.

1. Half-fill the base of a steamer with water, bring to the boil, then add the potatoes. Put the salmon in a steamer basket over the potatoes, season with salt and pepper, cover and cook for 8–10 minutes, or until the salmon flakes easily when pressed with a knife. Cook the potatoes for about 15 minutes, until tender.

2. Remove any skin from the salmon, then flake into chunky pieces, removing any bones.

3. Drain the potatoes and mash with the butter, then mix in the spring onions, lime zest, coriander, chilli, ginger and a little salt and pepper. Gently stir in the salmon. Dust a chopping board with the rice flour. Divide the salmon mixture into 8 mounds and pat into rounds on the chopping board. Chill for 15–30 minutes to firm up.

4. Meanwhile, make the chutney: heat the oil in a pan, add the garlic and fry for 2–3 minutes, until softened but not browned. Add the ginger, tomatoes, sugar and salt and pepper to taste, then simmer for about 5 minutes, stirring from time to time, until thickened. Remove from the heat and stir in the coriander.

5. To finish the fish cakes, preheat the oven to 200°C/400°F/ Gas Mark 6. Beat the eggs in a shallow dish. Put the breadcrumbs in another shallow dish. Dip each fish cake in egg and turn over with 2 forks, lift out and coat in the breadcrumbs.

6. Brush or spray a large baking sheet with oil, add the fish cakes and drizzle or spray a little extra oil on top. Bake for 20 minutes, turning after 10 minutes, until golden. Warm the chutney and serve with the fish cakes, with lime wedges and salad.

Freezing tip Open-freeze the fish cakes on a baking sheet at the end of step 5 until firm then wrap individually in clingfilm (plastic wrap), pack, seal and label. Freeze the chutney in an ice-cube tray until firm, then transfer the cubes to a plastic container, seal and label. Freeze fish cakes and chutney for up to 1 month. To serve, cook as many frozen fish cakes as you need, as in step 6, but for 30 minutes, until piping hot. Reheat as many cubes of chutney as you need in the microwave, until hot.

GF tip Gluten-free bread is expensive and goes stale quickly. Don't throw away leftover slices: instead, tear into pieces, including the crusts, and blitz in a blender or food processor to make breadcrumbs. Store in a resealable plastic bag in the freezer for up to 3 months.

OTHER FILLING IDEAS

• **Cheesy ham and egg crêpes** – make the spinach crêpe batter and cook just one side of each crêpe; as you turn it over to cook the second side, break an egg onto the cooked top of the crêpe. By the time the underside of the crêpe is done the egg will be cooked. Top each crêpe with 2 wafer-thin slices of ham, 1 heaped tbsp grated Cheddar or Gruyère cheese and a little of the reserved hot spinach. Fold and serve.

• **Brie and garlicky cherry tomato crêpes** – cut 200g/7oz cherry tomatoes in half and place in a foil-lined grill pan; sprinkle with 2 finely chopped garlic cloves and a little salt and pepper and drizzle with 1 tbsp olive oil. Grill for 5 minutes, until hot. Divide between the cooked spinach crêpes, top with the reserved hot spinach and 200g/7oz Brie cut into long thin slices. Fold and serve.

SPINACH AND SALMON
CRÊPES

SERVES 4

PREP: 20 MINUTES

COOK: 25 MINUTES

3 SALMON FILLETS, ABOUT 150g/5½oz EACH, SKINNED
SALT AND FRESHLY GROUND BLACK PEPPER
2–3 TBSP SUNFLOWER OIL
200g/7oz BABY SPINACH LEAVES, WASHED AND DRIED
150g/5½oz/⅔ CUP FULL-FAT CRÈME FRAÎCHE
FRESHLY GRATED PARMESAN CHEESE

Crêpes

85g/3oz/SCANT ¾ CUP FINE POLENTA (CORNMEAL)
85g/3oz/GENEROUS ½ CUP RICE FLOUR
PINCH OF GRATED NUTMEG
2 EGGS
2 TBSP FRESHLY GRATED PARMESAN CHEESE
200ml/7fl oz/GENEROUS ¾ CUP SEMI-SKIMMED
    (LOW-FAT) MILK

Cook's tip To save time, if you'd rather not grill fresh salmon, fill with strips of smoked salmon.

Bring back memories of French holidays with these delicate green-speckled crêpes filled with a luxurious spinach and salmon mix and finished with a sprinkling of Parmesan.

1. Preheat the grill (broiler). Line the grill rack with foil, lay the salmon on top and sprinkle with salt and pepper and a little oil. Grill for 10 minutes, turning once, until golden brown and the fish flakes when pressed with a knife. Wrap the foil around the fish and keep hot.

2. Meanwhile, cook the spinach in the microwave on high power for 2 minutes, or until just wilted.

3. Carefully measure out 55g/2oz of the spinach and place in a blender or food processor. Cover the rest of the spinach and keep hot. Add the crêpe ingredients to the blender or processor and blitz until smooth, then pour into a jug.

4. Heat a little oil in a medium sized non-stick frying pan over a medium-high heat, wipe off the excess with kitchen paper. Pour in a quarter of the crêpe mixture, tilt the pan to swirl the mixture into an even layer, then cook for a minute or two, until golden brown on the underside. Loosen the edges with a palette knife, flip over and cook the other side.

5. Slide the crêpe out onto a plate and keep hot while you make 3 more crêpes in the same way.

6. Put a crêpe on each of 4 serving plates. Spoon the remaining cooked spinach into the centre of each. Flake the salmon into pieces, discarding any skin and bones, then pile on top of the spinach. Spoon the crème fraîche over the salmon and sprinkle with a little grated Parmesan, salt and pepper. Fold two opposite edges in to the centre, then fold in the remaining two edges to make a square parcel and turn over so the joins are underneath. Sprinkle with a little extra Parmesan and serve immediately.

FRITTO MISTO

This light Mediterranean version of fish in batter is made with sea bass, squid, mussels and prawns, but the choice of fish is up to you. Try with small cubes of salmon, sliced squid, or a mix of fish and sliced vegetables. There's a fiery, garlicky pepper sauce for dunking.

SERVES 4
PREP: 15 MINUTES
COOK: 10–15 MINUTES

2 SEA BASS FILLETS, SKINNED AND
    CUT INTO BITE-SIZED PIECES
500g/1lb 2oz FROZEN MIXED SEAFOOD
    (SLICED SQUID, SHELLED MUSSELS AND PRAWNS/
    SHRIMP), DEFROSTED
JUICE OF ½ LEMON
1 LITRE/1¾ PINTS/4 CUPS SUNFLOWER OIL
    FOR DEEP-FRYING
LEMON WEDGES AND SALAD, TO SERVE

Batter

1 EGG WHITE
115g/4oz/SCANT 1 CUP TAPIOCA FLOUR
40g/1½oz/4 TBSP RICE FLOUR
1 TSP ROUGHLY CRUSHED PEPPERCORNS
LARGE PINCH OF SALT
1 EGG
150ml/5fl oz/⅔ CUP COLD WATER

Garlic and red pepper sauce

2 TBSP OLIVE OIL
1 ONION, FINELY CHOPPED
1 RED PEPPER, CORED, DESEEDED AND DICED
3 GARLIC CLOVES, FINELY CHOPPED
LARGE PINCH OF DRIED CHILLI FLAKES
¼ TSP SMOKED HOT PAPRIKA
JUICE OF ½ LEMON
SALT AND FRESHLY GROUND BLACK PEPPER

1. First, make the sauce: heat the oil in a saucepan, add the onion and red pepper and cook for 5 minutes, until softened. Add the garlic and cook for 3–4 minutes, until softened. Stir in the chilli flakes and paprika and cook for a few seconds, then mix in the lemon juice and plenty of salt and pepper. Whizz in a blender until smooth, then spoon into a serving dish.

2. Rinse the fish and seafood with cold water, drain well and pat dry with kitchen paper. Toss in the lemon juice.

3. To make the batter, whisk the egg white in a small clean glass bowl until soft peaks form. Mix the flours, peppercorns and salt in another bowl, add the whole egg and water and whisk together until smooth, then fold in the egg white.

4. Half-fill a deep saucepan with the oil and heat to 190°C/375°F, or until a cube of bread browns in 20 seconds. Dip the fish and seafood into the batter, a few pieces at a time, then lift out with a slotted spoon and drop into the oil. Cook for about 3 minutes, until the batter is bubbly and pale golden.

5. Lift out with a slotted spoon and drain on kitchen paper. Continue dipping and frying until all the fish is cooked. Serve with spoonfuls of the sauce, lemon wedges and salad.

Cook's tips

This light bubbly batter can also be used to coat larger pieces of fish for more traditional British fish and chips. For deep-frying, reduce the heat to 180°C/350°F, or until a cube of bread browns in 30 seconds, as the pieces of fish will take longer to cook.

For fans of tempura, use the batter to coat slices of courgette (zucchini), mushrooms, asparagus and prawns (shrimp) and serve with gluten-free soy sauce flavoured with a little chilli.

For salt and pepper squid, dip thinly sliced squid into the batter, deep-fry until crisp, drain and serve with sweet and sour plum chutney, on a bed of salad leaves.

ONION AND CAULIFLOWER BHAJIS

MAKES ABOUT 16
PREP: 15 MINUTES
COOK: 10–15 MINUTES

115g/4oz/1¼ CUPS GRAM (CHICKPEA) FLOUR
55g/2oz/6 TBSP RICE FLOUR
¼ TSP SALT
½ TSP TURMERIC
½ TSP GROUND CORIANDER
¼ TSP CHILLI POWDER
1 TSP CUMIN SEEDS, ROUGHLY CRUSHED
2.5CM/1IN PIECE OF FRESH GINGER,
    PEELED AND GRATED
2 GARLIC CLOVES, FINELY CHOPPED
200ml/7fl oz/GENEROUS ¾ CUP COLD WATER
½ CAULIFLOWER, CUT INTO SMALL FLORETS,
    THEN SLICED
2 ONIONS, THINLY SLICED
1 LITRE/1¾ PINTS/4 CUPS SUNFLOWER OIL
    FOR DEEP-FRYING

Coriander and ginger dip

150g/5½oz/⅔ CUP PLAIN YOGURT
2CM/¾IN PIECE OF FRESH GINGER,
    PEELED AND GRATED
SMALL HANDFUL OF FRESH CORIANDER (CILANTRO) LEAVES
SALT AND FRESHLY GROUND BLACK PEPPER

Quick and easy to make, these are great served as a nibble with drinks before your favourite curry. You might like to try your own veggie mixes: sliced mushrooms and green beans work well, or sliced courgettes (zucchini) or green peppers.

1. To make the dip, put all the ingredients into a blender and blend until smooth, then spoon into a serving dish.

2. To make the bhajis, sift the flours, salt and ground spices into a mixing bowl, stir in the cumin seeds, ginger and garlic, then whisk in the water to make a smooth batter. Add the cauliflower and onions and toss gently in the batter.

3. Heat the oil in a large saucepan to 180–190°C/ 350–375°F, or until a cube of bread browns in 30 seconds. Carefully drop heaped dessertspoonfuls of the onion and cauliflower mixture into the hot oil until 4 or 5 bhajis are in the pan. Cook for about 3 minutes, until golden brown.

4. Lift out with a slotted spoon and drain on kitchen paper. Continue deep-frying the bhajis in batches until all the mixture has been used. Serve warm with the coriander and ginger dip.

GF tip Don't be tempted to reuse oil that has been used to deep-fry wheat- or gluten-containing foods as these will contaminate the oil.

SPINACH AND POTATO
SAMOSAS

MAKES 16

PREP: 1 HOUR

COOK: 35 MINUTES

Filling

350g/12oz POTATOES, SCRUBBED

1 TBSP SUNFLOWER OIL

1 ONION, FINELY CHOPPED

½ TSP BLACK MUSTARD SEEDS

1 TSP CUMIN SEEDS, ROUGHLY CRUSHED

1–2 SMALL GREEN CHILLIES, DESEEDED AND THINLY SLICED

1 TSP TURMERIC

1 TSP GROUND CORIANDER

SALT

85g/3oz/GENEROUS ½ CUP FROZEN PEAS

55g/2oz FRESH SPINACH, SLICED

SMALL HANDFUL OF CHOPPED FRESH CORIANDER (CILANTRO)

Pastry

175g/6oz/SCANT 1 CUP GRAM (CHICKPEA) FLOUR

55g/2oz/6 TBSP RICE FLOUR, PLUS EXTRA FOR DUSTING

½ TSP XANTHAN GUM

25g/1oz/2 TBSP UNSALTED BUTTER OR GHEE, MELTED

6 TBSP COLD WATER

1 LITRE/1¾ PINTS/4 CUPS SUNFLOWER OR VEGETABLE OIL FOR DEEP-FRYING

Freezing tip Pack cooked samosas in a plastic container and freeze for up to 1 month. Reheat wrapped in foil at 190°C/375°F/Gas Mark 5 for 15-20 minutes or until hot through, check and cut one in half before serving.

These bite-sized Indian pastries are a little fiddly to make, but they can be prepared in advance and then cooked just before serving.

1. To make the filling, boil the potatoes in their skins for about 20 minutes, until tender. Drain, rinse with cold water until cool enough to handle, then scrape away the skins with a small knife. Cut the potatoes into small dice and set aside.

2. Heat the oil in a frying pan over a low heat, add the onion, mustard and cumin seeds and cook gently for 5 minutes, or until just beginning to colour. Stir in the chillies, turmeric, ground coriander and salt, then add the peas, spinach and fresh coriander and cook for a few minutes, until the peas have just thawed and the spinach just wilted. Remove from the heat, stir in the potatoes and leave to cool.

3. To make the pastry, sift the flours, ¼ tsp salt and the xanthan gum into a bowl. Add the melted butter or ghee, then mix in enough of the cold water to make a soft but not sticky dough.

4. Cut the dough into 8 pieces; loosely cover 7 of the pieces with clingfilm (plastic wrap) so that they don't dry out. Roll out the first piece between 2 sheets of baking parchment, lightly dusted with rice flour, to form a circle about 15cm/6in in diameter. Turn the dough from time to time to prevent it sticking.

5. Cut the circle in half, brush the edges of each semi-circle with water, and spoon a little of the filling into the centre of each, then fold each one into a cone shape by folding the dough up from the tip of a long straight edge, bringing the cut edge up and over the filling, then doing the same with the other straight edge. Fold over the top curved edge of the cone and pinch the edges together to seal well. Transfer to a baking sheet lined with baking parchment and repeat until you have made 16 samosas.

6. To cook, half-fill a large saucepan with oil. Heat to 180–190°C/350–375°F, or until a cube of bread browns in 30 seconds. Cook the samosas in batches for 3–4 minutes, until golden brown, then lift out with a slotted spoon and drain on kitchen paper. Serve warm.

CHEESY LEEK GRIDDLE CAKES

MAKES 8
PREP: 15 MINUTES
COOK: ABOUT 20 MINUTES

1 TBSP OLIVE OIL, PLUS EXTRA FOR COOKING THE CAKES
115g/4oz LEEK, THINLY SLICED
55g/2oz/4 TBSP UNSALTED BUTTER
115g/4oz/¾ CUP POTATO FLOUR
115g/4oz/¾ CUP RICE FLOUR,
    PLUS EXTRA FOR DUSTING
1 TSP GLUTEN-FREE BAKING POWDER
115g/4oz GRUYÈRE OR CHEDDAR CHEESE, GRATED
SALT AND FRESHLY GROUND BLACK PEPPER
1 EGG, BEATEN
6–8 TBSP SEMI-SKIMMED (LOW-FAT) MILK

These are quick and easy to make for a Sunday brunch or midweek supper – and as they are cooked in a frying pan, there's no need to turn on the oven. They are delicious served with a poached egg and just-wilted spinach, grilled bacon, or baked beans, or spread with a little butter and serve alongside a bowl of soup.

1. Heat the oil in a frying pan, add the leek and cook gently for 5 minutes, until softened. Take the pan off the heat, add the butter and stir until melted.

2. Put the flours and baking powder into a mixing bowl, add the cheese and a little salt and pepper and stir together. Add the leek and butter, then the egg. Gradually mix in enough milk to make a soft but not sticky dough.

3. Cut the dough in half. On a chopping board or a piece of baking parchment dusted with a little rice flour, lightly roll out or pat half of the dough to form a 15cm/6in circle. Cut into 4 wedges.

4. Reheat the frying pan over a medium heat, add the 4 potato cakes and cook for 8 minutes, turning once or twice, until golden. Meanwhile, roll out the remaining dough to make 4 more potato wedges. Lift out the cooked cakes, wrap in a clean teacloth to keep warm, and cook the remaining cakes in the same way, adding a little extra oil if needed. Serve hot.

GF tip Potato flour has a short shelf life, so buy in small quantities. Griddle cakes are traditionally made with freshly cooked and mashed potatoes with the addition of wheat flour, but potato flour makes a quick alternative. Don't confuse it with the more refined potato starch, which can be used to thicken sauces and soups, or in cakes if mixed with other gluten-free flours.

CINNAMON PANCAKES
WITH BLUEBERRY COMPOTE

SERVES 4
PREP: 25 MINUTES
COOK: 15 MINUTES

40g/1½oz/6 TBSP FINE POLENTA (CORNMEAL)
40g/1½oz/5 TBSP TAPIOCA FLOUR
LARGE PINCH OF GROUND CINNAMON
1 TSP BICARBONATE OF SODA (BAKING SODA)
1 EGG
200g/7oz/GENEROUS ¾ CUP LOW-FAT PLAIN YOGURT,
    PLUS EXTRA TO SERVE
4 TBSP COLD WATER
2 TBSP SUNFLOWER OR VEGETABLE OIL
GROUND CINNAMON, TO SERVE

Blueberry compote

3 TBSP CASTER (SUPERFINE) SUGAR
2 TSP GLUTEN-FREE CORNFLOUR (CORNSTARCH)
JUICE OF ½ LEMON
200g/7oz/1⅓ CUPS BLUEBERRIES

A change from toast for breakfast, these American-style thick pancakes can be made in minutes and topped with a warm blueberry compote and spoonfuls of yogurt. Alternatively, top with another fruit compote, sliced bananas and maple syrup, or grilled fresh apricots with honey and cinnamon.

1. To make the compote, mix the sugar and cornflour together in a small saucepan and stir in the lemon juice to make a paste. Add the blueberries and cook over a gentle heat, stirring from time to time, until the blueberries soften and the juices thicken.

2. To make the pancakes, mix the polenta, tapioca flour, cinnamon and bicarbonate of soda together in a bowl. Add the egg, yogurt and water and mix to a smooth, thick batter.

3. Pour a little oil into a large frying pan, wipe off the excess with kitchen paper, then heat the pan over a medium heat. Add heaped tablespoons of the pancake batter, leaving a little space between each spoonful and cook until the underside is golden and bubbles are just beginning to appear on the surface.

4. Turn the pancakes over and cook the second side. Scoop out of the pan and wrap in a clean teacloth to keep warm. Wipe the pan with a little more oil and kitchen paper and continue making pancakes until all the mixture has been used.

5. Serve the pancakes on warmed plates, spoon the warm compote over the top and serve with spoonfuls of yogurt with a dusting of cinnamon.

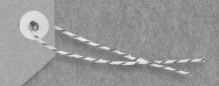

GF tip While it is tempting to swap different gluten-free flours one for the other (especially if you have run out of one type), remember that some have quite different textures and may need extra liquid to compensate.

GF tip Polenta comes in different grades, from fine to coarse; choose the finest for the smoothest texture.

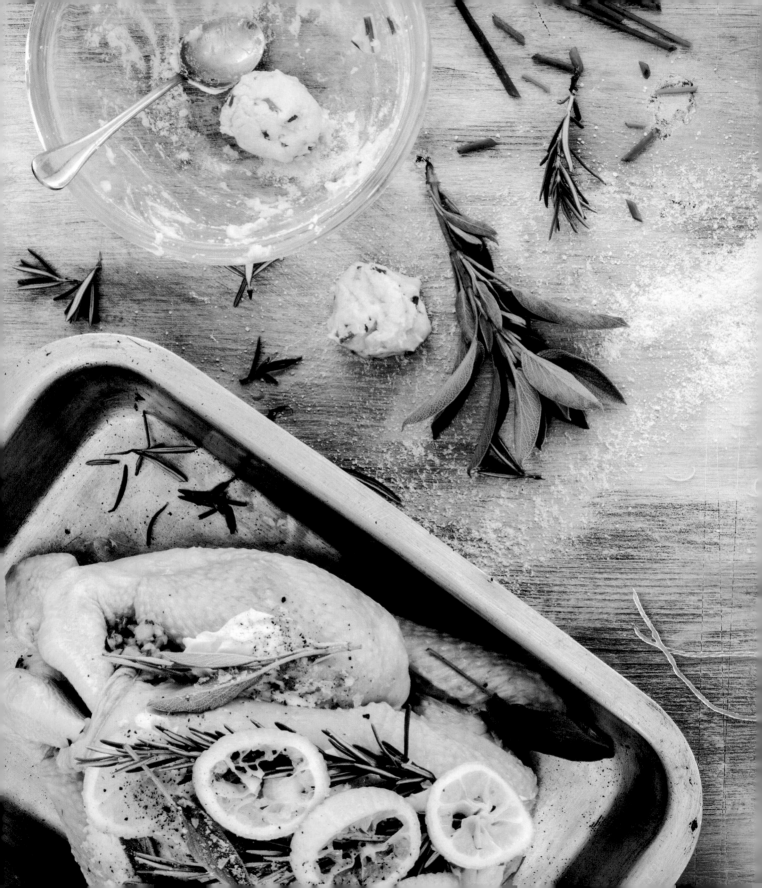

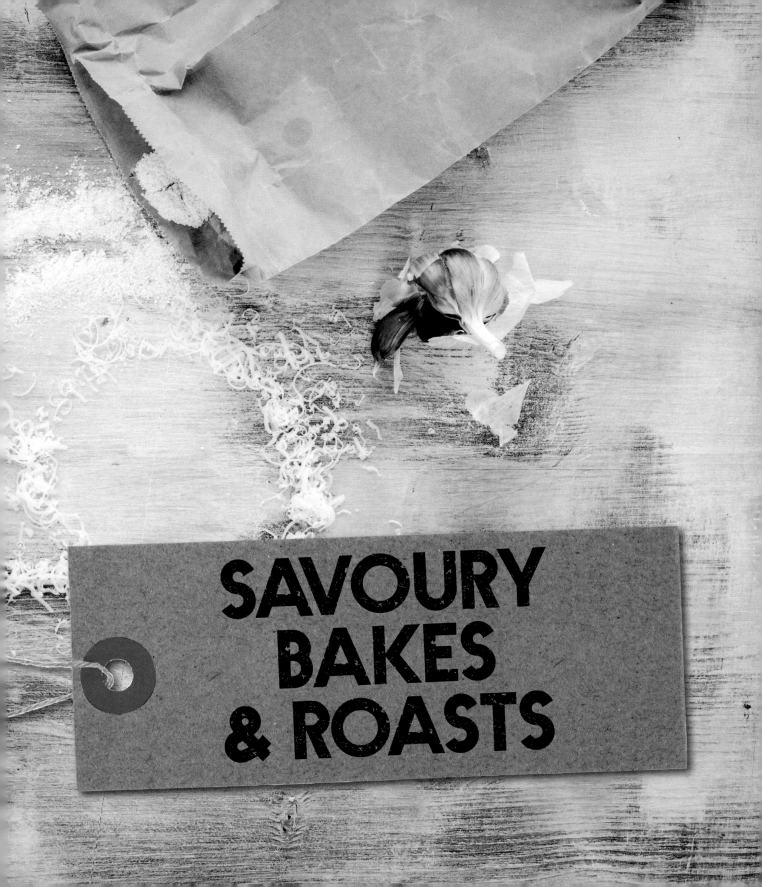

SAVOURY BAKES & ROASTS

SAVOURY BAKES & ROASTS

From weekday suppers to a Sunday roast, when it comes to eating gluten-free, the devil is in the detail. How do you thicken your sauce or gravy? What about bread-based stuffings and meatloaf? Can you adapt dumplings and cobbler toppings? Fortunately, there are plenty of solutions.

Casseroles can be thickened with rice flour instead of wheat flour: either stir the flour into the fried onions before adding stock at the beginning of cooking, or add at the end of cooking as *beurre manié*, where a little rice flour and butter are mixed to a paste and whisked into the casserole in small pieces. A teaspoon or two of cornflour mixed with a little water can also be stirred into the sauce at the end, brought back to the boil and stirred until thickened. For meat or bean mixtures cooked on the stove top you may find that the sauce needs no added thickening because the liquid evaporates as it simmers, resulting in a thick, concentrated sauce. The same goes for gravy and pan sauces – you can speed up the evaporation by boiling the liquid rapidly, a process known as reduction.

A casserole is perfect for a homely supper that can be left to cook in the oven while you get on with something else. Add polenta and tapioca dumplings (page 50), or a cobbler topping made with chestnut flour (page 52). Alternatively, add a hotpot-style layer of thinly sliced potatoes just before the casserole goes in the oven, or serve with a spoonful of mashed potato instead.

Roast chicken with all the trimmings needn't be off the menu. You can make stuffings with gluten-free breadcrumbs, or use mashed chickpeas as a base (page 54).

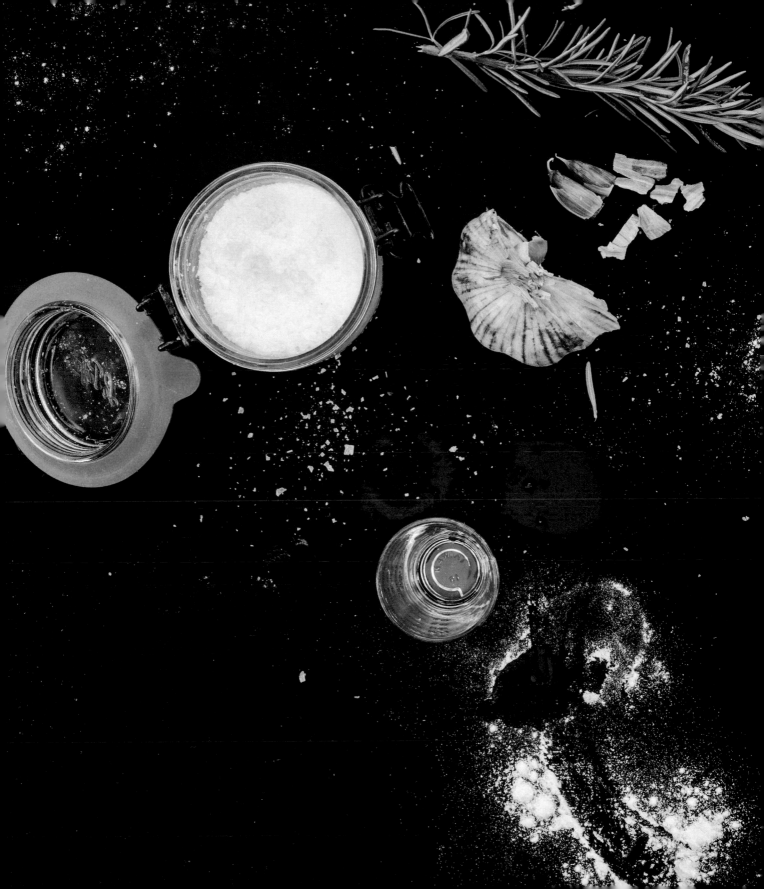

BEEF
CARBONNADE
WITH CHIVE DUMPLINGS

SERVES 4

PREP: 30 MINUTES

COOK: 2½ HOURS

2 TBSP SUNFLOWER OIL

800g/1lb 12oz LEAN STEWING BEEF,
    FAT TRIMMED OFF, BEEF CUBED

2 SLICES OF BACK BACON, DICED

400g/14oz SHALLOTS, PEELED, HALVED IF LARGE

2 TBSP RICE FLOUR

500ml/18fl oz/2¼ CUPS GLUTEN-FREE BEER

300ml/10fl oz/1¼ CUPS GLUTEN-FREE BEEF STOCK

2 TBSP LIGHT MUSCOVADO (BROWN) SUGAR

2 BAY LEAVES

1 TBSP WHITE MUSTARD SEEDS, ROUGHLY CRUSHED

SALT AND FRESHLY GROUND BLACK PEPPER

3 CELERY STALKS, THICKLY SLICED

500g/1lb 2oz CHANTENAY CARROTS, HALVED IF LARGE

Dumplings

115g/4oz FINE POLENTA (CORNMEAL)

55g/2oz/½ CUP TAPIOCA FLOUR

1 TSP GLUTEN-FREE BAKING POWDER

85g/3oz WHITE VEGETABLE FAT, DICED

SMALL HANDFUL OF FRESH CHIVES, SNIPPED

ABOUT 6 TBSP COLD WATER

A comforting stew to banish the winter blues, carbonnade originates in Belgium and is made with beer – in this case, gluten-free beer. Ladle into shallow soup bowls and enjoy curled up on the sofa while you watch a favourite film.

1. Preheat the oven to 180°C/350°F/Gas Mark 4. Heat the oil in a large frying pan, add the beef, a few pieces at a time, and fry over a high heat until browned, in batches if necessary to avoid overcrowding the pan. Scoop out of the pan with a slotted spoon and transfer to a large casserole dish.

2. Add the bacon and shallots to the pan juices and cook over a medium heat until the bacon is just beginning to turn golden. Sprinkle the flour over and stir in. Add the beer, stock, sugar, bay leaves and mustard and season generously with salt and pepper. Bring to the boil.

3. Add the celery and carrots to the beef, then pour over the beery bacon mixture. Cover and cook in the oven for 2 hours, or until the beef is tender.

4. To make the dumplings, sift the polenta, tapioca flour and baking powder into a bowl. Add the fat and rub in until it forms fine crumbs. Stir in the chives and season generously with salt and pepper, then gradually mix in enough water to form a soft dough.

5. Scoop 12 spoonfuls on to a board, roll each into a ball and drop into the hot beef casserole, replace the lid and return to the oven for about 20 minutes, until the dumplings are cooked through. Spoon into shallow bowls and serve.

GF tip Shredded suet is often sold dusted with wheat flour to stop the pieces of fat sticking together. Gluten-free shredded suet is available, but if you can't find it, white vegetable fat, used mainly for pastry making, is a useful alternative.

Freezing tip The beef stew (without the dumplings) can be frozen in a plastic bag for up to 3 months. Thaw overnight in the fridge. Reheat the stew until piping hot through, then drop in the dumplings and cook as in step 5.

GF tip Most beers, including lager, stout and ale, are made with barley, which contains gluten. Happily, gluten-free beers made with sorghum, buckwheat and rice are becoming more widely available from artisan microbrewers and larger supermarkets. Look online for stockists near you. Alternatively, just use extra stock – or part red wine, part stock.

LAMB AND CHESTNUT
COBBLER

SERVES 4–6

PREP: 25 MINUTES

COOK: 2½–3 HOURS

2 TBSP OLIVE OIL

3 LAMB SHANKS, WEIGHING ABOUT 1.25kg/2lb 12oz

1 LARGE ONION, FINELY CHOPPED

250g/9oz FLAT MUSHROOMS, THICKLY SLICED

2 GARLIC CLOVES, FINELY CHOPPED

450ml/16fl oz/2 CUPS GLUTEN-FREE LAMB STOCK

400g CAN CHOPPED TOMATOES

200g/7oz VACUUM-PACKED PREPARED CHESTNUTS

2 BAY LEAVES

½ TSP GROUND CINNAMON

SALT AND FRESHLY GROUND BLACK PEPPER

Cobbler topping

175g/6oz CHESTNUT FLOUR

115g/4oz/SCANT 1 CUP TAPIOCA FLOUR,
    PLUS EXTRA FOR DUSTING

1 TSP XANTHAN GUM

2 TSP GLUTEN-FREE BAKING POWDER

¼ TSP GROUND CINNAMON

85g/3oz/6 TBSP UNSALTED BUTTER, DICED

1 EGG

100ml/3½fl oz/ ½ cup SEMI-SKIMMED (LOW-FAT) MILK

GF tip Chestnut flour is a fine flour with a wonderful nutty sweetness. It is more expensive than some other flours and is sold in larger health food shops, as well as online.

A slow-cooked autumnal recipe that won't come to much harm if you leave it in the oven for another half hour or so. The casserole base can be made a day ahead, or frozen. All it needs to accompany it is a simple green vegetable, such as baby Brussels sprouts or Savoy cabbage.

1. Preheat the oven to 160°C/325°F/Gas Mark 3. Heat 1 tbsp oil in a large flameproof casserole over a medium–high heat, add the lamb shanks and cook for 10 minutes, turning until evenly browned. Lift out onto a plate. Add the remaining oil and the onion and cook for 5 minutes, or until softened.

2. Stir in the mushrooms and garlic and cook for 2 minutes, then pour in the stock and tomatoes. Add the chestnuts, bay leaves and cinnamon and season generously with salt and pepper. Return the lamb to the casserole and bring to the boil.

3. Cover and transfer to the oven for 2–2½ hours, or until the lamb is very tender.

4. Lift the lamb out of the casserole onto a chopping board. Using a knife and fork, peel away the skin and remove the bones. Cut the meat into bite-sized pieces, return to the casserole and put back in the oven with the lid on.

5. To make the cobbler topping, put the flours, xanthan gum, baking powder, cinnamon and some salt and pepper into a bowl and mix well. Add the butter and rub in until it forms fine crumbs. Add the egg, reserving a little bit for glazing, then gradually mix in enough milk to make a soft but not sticky dough (you won't need all the milk).

6. Tip the dough onto a chopping board dusted with a little tapioca flour. Use your hands to pat the dough out to form a circle slightly smaller than the top of the casserole and about 2cm/¾in thick. Cut into 8 wedges.

7. Take the casserole out of the oven and increase the oven temperature to 190°C/375°F/Gas Mark 5. Arrange the cobbler wedges on top of the casserole, brush lightly with the remaining egg and milk and bake for 15–20 minutes, until the topping is browned and well risen. Spoon into bowls and serve with a cooked green vegetable.

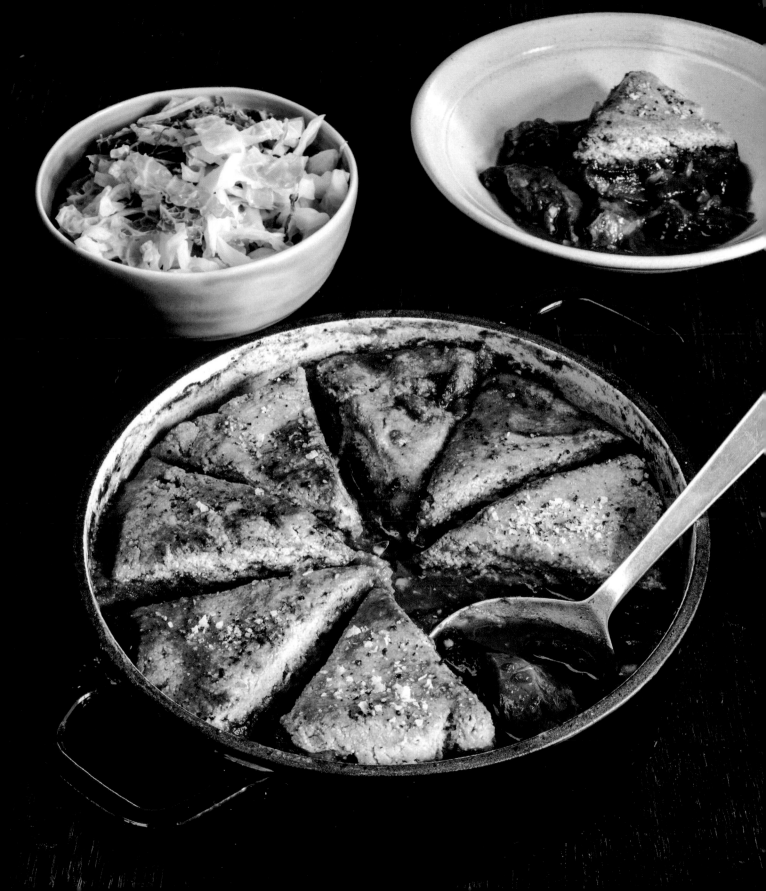

ROAST CHICKEN

SERVES 4
PREP: 25 MINUTES
COOK: 1 HOUR 40 MINUTES

1 CHICKEN, WEIGHING ABOUT 1.8kg/4lb
25g/1oz/2 TBSP UNSALTED BUTTER, SOFTENED
1 TBSP SUNFLOWER OIL

Lemon and herb stuffing

1 TBSP SUNFLOWER OIL
1 ONION, FINELY CHOPPED
400g/14oz CANNED CHICKPEAS, DRAINED
4 SPRIGS OF FRESH SAGE
4 SPRIGS OF FRESH ROSEMARY
SMALL BUNCH OF MIXED FRESH PARSLEY AND CHIVES
1 UNWAXED LEMON, GRATED ZEST AND JUICE
1 EGG, BEATEN
SALT AND FRESHLY GROUND BLACK PEPPER

Gravy

450ml/16fl oz/2 CUPS GLUTEN-FREE CHICKEN STOCK
4 TBSP DRY SHERRY

Cook's tip If you prefer a thicker gravy, mix 1 tbsp cornflour with a little water to make a smooth paste. Stir into the hot gravy, simmer until thickened, then strain into a jug.

All the family loves roast chicken and with a few easy tweaks it becomes a gluten-free meal. Chickpeas replace bread in a herby stuffing.

1. Preheat the oven to 190°C/375°F/Gas Mark 5.

2. To make the stuffing, heat the oil in a frying pan, add the onion and cook for 5 minutes, until softened and just beginning to brown.

3. Put the chickpeas in a food processor and blitz to a coarse mash, or mash in a bowl if preferred. Chop the leaves of 2 sprigs of sage and rosemary, add to the chickpeas with the chopped fresh herbs, zest and juice of the lemon and beaten egg. Stir in the fried onion and plenty of salt and pepper. Cut the lemon skin into thin slices.

4. Put the chicken into a roasting pan. Spoon the stuffing into the body cavity of the chicken. Season the outside of the chicken, spread with the butter, drizzle with the oil, then place the remaining sage and rosemary sprigs over the chicken breast. Top with the sliced lemon, then loosely wrap in foil.

5. Roast for 1 hour. Remove the foil and baste with the pan juices. Return to the oven and roast for 40 minutes without the foil, until the chicken is a deep golden colour and the juices run clear when the chicken is pierced through the thickest part of the leg. Transfer the chicken to a serving plate.

6. To make the gravy, pour off most of the fat from the roasting pan to leave about 2–3 tbsp of meat juices. Add the stock, sherry and a little salt and pepper to taste. Bring to the boil, scraping up the pan juices, boil for about 2 minutes, until slightly thickened, then strain into a serving jug.

Recipe continues...

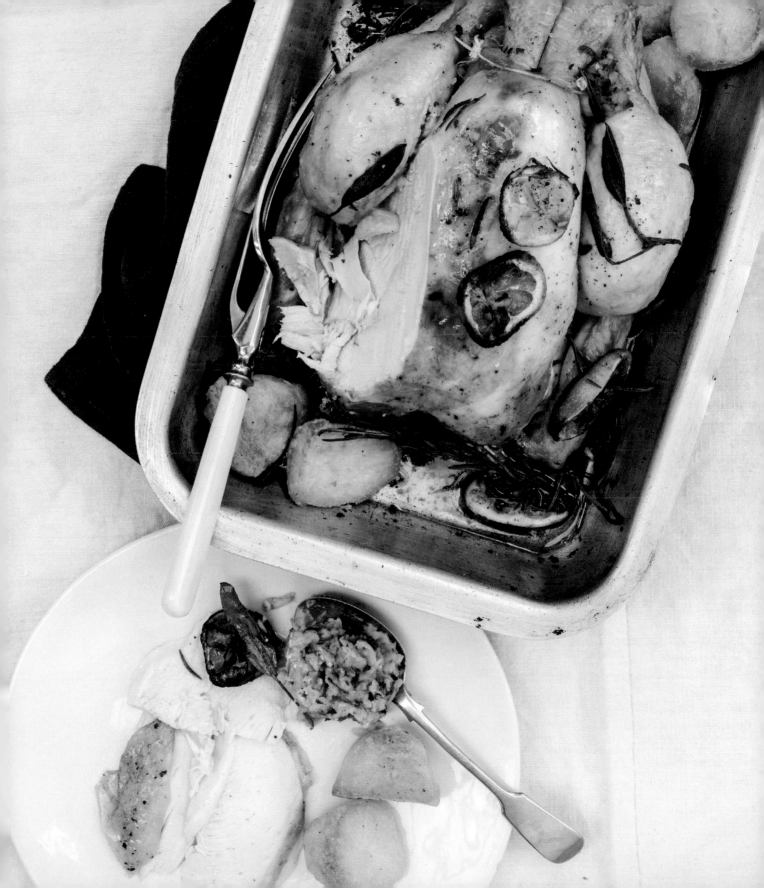

ROAST CHICKEN
...CONTINUED

EXTRA CRUNCHY
ROAST POTATOES

SERVES 4

PREP: 10 MINUTES

COOK: 45 MINUTES

Peel 700g/1lb 9oz baking potatoes and cut into chunky 5cm/2in pieces. Add to a saucepan of boiling water and par-boil for 10 minutes. Drain into a colander and shake the colander to roughen the edges of the potatoes, then sprinkle with 2 tbsp fine polenta (cornmeal). Heat 4 tbsp olive or sunflower oil in a roasting pan on the shelf above the chicken for 5 minutes. Spoon the potatoes into the hot roasting pan, baste the tops with some of the oil, then roast for about 40 minutes, turning once or twice until golden brown. Drain well and serve with the roast chicken.

GF tip Stock cubes and cornflour are not always gluten-free: check the labels before you buy.

BACON, LEEK AND
TARRAGON STUFFING

SERVES 4

PREP: 10 MINUTES

Chop 2 slices of smoked streaky bacon and cook in a dry frying pan until just beginning to colour. Add 1 small chopped leek and 1 tbsp olive oil and cook for 2–3 minutes, until the leeks have just softened. Drain a 400g can of chickpeas, mash, then stir in the leek mixture, 1 chopped tarragon sprig, 1 egg and salt and pepper.

Spoon the stuffing into the chicken, spread with 25g/1oz butter, 1 tbsp oil and salt and pepper. Add 2 sprigs of tarragon and cover with 4 slices of smoked streaky bacon. Loosely cover with foil and cook as in the recipe on page 54.

SUN-DRIED TOMATO
AND GARLIC STUFFING

SERVES 4

PREP: 10 MINUTES

Fry 1 chopped onion in 1 tbsp olive oil, until softened. Add 2 finely chopped garlic cloves and 40g/1½oz spinach and cook for 1 minute, until the spinach has just wilted. Drain a 400g can of chickpeas, mash, then stir in the spinach mixture, 40g/1½oz chopped sun-dried tomatoes, 1 egg and salt and pepper.

Spoon the stuffing into the chicken, spread with 25g/1oz butter, 1 tbsp oil and salt and pepper plus a little paprika. Add a halved garlic bulb to the roasting pan, cover with foil and cook as as in the recipe on page 54.

BOBOTIE

SERVES 4
PREP: 20 MINUTES
COOK: 45–50 MINUTES

🍽✹

1 TBSP SUNFLOWER OIL
500g/1lb 2oz EXTRA-LEAN MINCED (GROUND) BEEF
1 ONION, FINELY CHOPPED
2 GARLIC CLOVES, FINELY CHOPPED
4 TSP MEDIUM-HOT CURRY POWDER,
    PLUS EXTRA FOR THE TOPPING
1 TBSP APRICOT JAM
1 TBSP TOMATO PUREE (TOMATO PASTE)
2 TBSP RED WINE VINEGAR
1 CARROT, GRATED
1 SMALL BANANA, PEELED AND DICED
3 TBSP RAISINS
55g/2oz/5 TBSP RED LENTILS
SALT AND FRESHLY GROUND BLACK PEPPER
4 BAY LEAVES
2 EGGS
200ml/7fl oz/GENEROUS ¾ CUP SEMI-SKIMMED
    (LOW-FAT) MILK

Cook's tip Don't be put off by the idea of adding bananas and raisins to minced beef: they add a gentle sweetness that balances the vinegar and adds depth of flavour.

This South African meatloaf is traditionally made with milk-soaked bread: red lentils offer a tasty gluten-free alternative. Serve hot with spiced yellow rice (boiled with a pinch of turmeric) and tomato and onion salad, or cold for lunch next day.

1. Preheat the oven to 180°C/350°F/Gas Mark 4. Heat the oil in a frying pan over a medium-high heat, add the beef and onion and fry for 5 minutes, stirring and breaking up the meat with a spoon until it is evenly browned and the onion is just beginning to colour.

2. Stir in the garlic, curry powder, jam, tomato purée and vinegar, then mix in the carrot, banana, raisins and lentils. Season with salt and pepper to taste, then press into a 1.4 litre/2½ pint rectangular ovenproof dish (about 5cm/2in deep) and smooth the top.

3. Arrange the bay leaves on top of the mixture. Beat the eggs and milk together with a large pinch of curry powder and a little salt and pepper, then pour over the bay leaves. Bake for 40–45 minutes, until the custard topping is set and golden and the meat is cooked through. Check after 30 minutes and loosely cover the top with foil if it seems to be browning too quickly.

4. Leave to cool for 15 minutes, then cut into thick slices and serve with boiled rice and a tomato and red onion salad or green salad.

CHEESE SOUFFLÉ
WITH CIDERED APPLES

SERVES 4

PREP: 30 MINUTES

COOK: 17–20 MINUTES

70g/2½oz/5 TBSP UNSALTED BUTTER
55g/2oz PARMESAN CHEESE, FINELY GRATED
115g/4oz GRUYÈRE OR CHEDDAR CHEESE, FINELY GRATED
25g/1oz/3 TBSP FINE POLENTA (CORNMEAL)
25g/1oz/2 TBSP RICE FLOUR
300ml/10fl oz/1¼ CUPS SEMI-SKIMMED (LOW-FAT) MILK
1 TSP GLUTEN-FREE MUSTARD POWDER,
    SUCH AS COLMAN'S
SALT AND CAYENNE PEPPER
4 EGGS, SEPARATED
WATERCRESS, TO SERVE

Cidered apples

25g/1oz/2 TBSP UNSALTED BUTTER
3 DESSERT APPLES, CORED AND DICED
1 TBSP CASTER (SUPERFINE) SUGAR
1 TBSP CIDER VINEGAR
4 TBSP COLD WATER

Soufflés aren't difficult to make: the crucial thing is to get everyone sitting at the table before you take the soufflé out of the oven. The parchment and string are not essential, but they will stop any overspills as the soufflé rises and add theatre when you snip the string and peel away the paper to reveal a gravity-defying soufflé, even if only for a few minutes.

1. Preheat the oven to 190°C/375°F/Gas Mark 5. Use some of the measured butter to generously grease 4 individual soufflé dishes (10cm/4in in diameter and 6cm/2½in tall). Mix the cheeses together, then sprinkle a generous tablespoon into each soufflé dish, turning to coat the base and sides evenly.

2. Wrap a double thickness strip of baking parchment around the side of each soufflé dish, so that the paper stands about 4cm/1½in above the top, and tie in place with string. Put the dishes on a baking sheet.

3. Melt the remaining butter in a saucepan, stir in the polenta and rice flour, then gradually mix in the milk and bring to the boil, stirring until thickened and smooth. Remove from the heat and stir in the remaining cheeses, mustard and plenty of salt and pepper, then the egg yolks. Leave to cool for 10 minutes.

4. Whisk the egg whites in a large clean, glass bowl until soft peaks form. Fold a large spoonful into the cheese mixture to loosen it slightly, then fold in the remaining egg whites. Divide the mixture among the soufflé dishes. Bake for 17–20 minutes, or until well risen, the tops are deep golden brown and the centres are still slightly soft.

5. Meanwhile, make the cidered apples. Melt the butter in a frying pan over a medium heat, add the apples and fry for 2–3 minutes, until just beginning to soften. Add the sugar, vinegar and water and simmer until the juices are syrupy.

6. As soon as the soufflés are ready, transfer the dishes to serving plates, add some watercress and a spoonful of the apples. Snip the string, peel off the parchment and serve immediately.

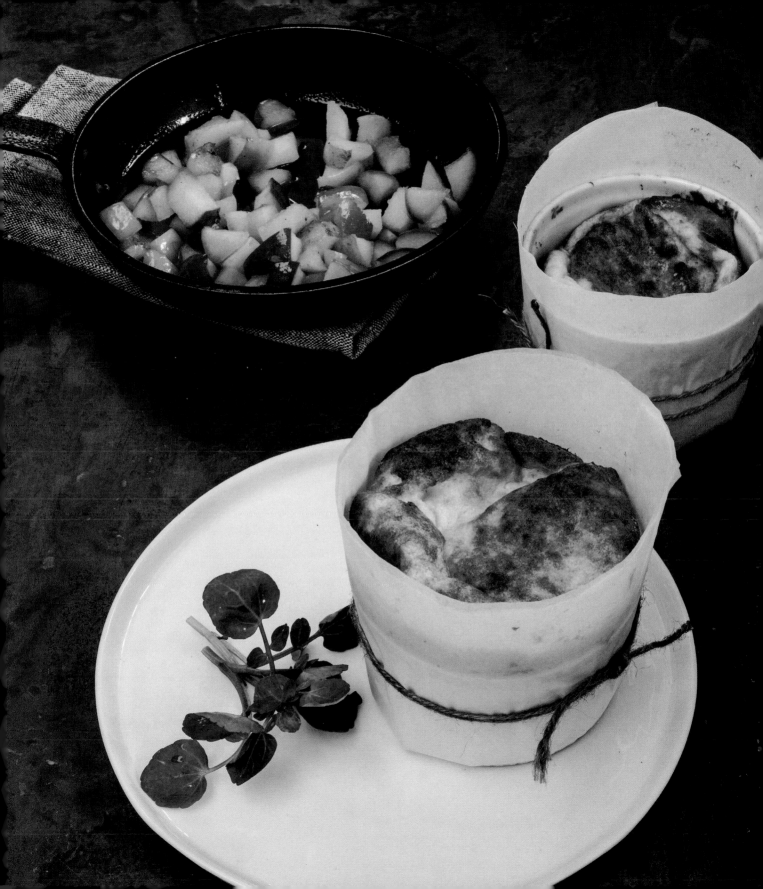

Cook's tips

This mixture can also be cooked in a 15cm/6in diameter (9cm/3½in tall) soufflé dish for 25–30 minutes.

You might like to add other ingredients to the cheese mixture in step 3: 1 large sliced and slowly fried onion; a handful of garlicky fried and sliced mushrooms; a handful of toasted and roughly chopped hazelnuts; or some chopped herbs.

VARIATIONS

• **Smoked salmon and dill soufflé** – omit the cheese and mustard. Fold 4 tbsp full-fat crème fraîche, 3 tbsp chopped fresh dill and the grated zest of 1 unwaxed lemon into the mixture at step 3. Fold in 100g/3½oz chopped smoked salmon just before folding in the whisked egg whites at step 4. Bake as on page 58.

• **Blue cheese and rocket soufflé** – omit the Gruyère or Cheddar cheese. Stir in 150g/5½oz blue cheese, crumbled into small pieces, at step 3. Fold in 25g/1oz chopped rocket (arugula) leaves just before folding in the whisked egg whites at step 4. Bake as on page 58.

BEETROOT
AND BLACK BEAN
CHILLI

SERVES 4	
PREP: 20 MINUTES	
COOK: 35–40 MINUTES	

1–2 SMALL DRIED CHIPOTLE CHILLIES
1 TBSP SUNFLOWER OIL
1 LARGE ONION, CHOPPED
2 RED PEPPERS, QUARTERED, CORED AND DESEEDED
1 BUNCH (ABOUT 5) BEETROOT (BEETS), TRIMMED, PEELED
    AND CUBED
2 GARLIC CLOVES, FINELY CHOPPED
½ TSP CUMIN SEEDS
½ TSP GROUND CLOVES
400g CAN BLACK BEANS, RINSED AND DRAINED
400g CAN CHOPPED TOMATOES
300ml/10fl oz/1¼ CUPS GLUTEN-FREE VEGETABLE STOCK
2 TBSP DARK MUSCOVADO (BROWN) SUGAR
2 BAY LEAVES
1 TSP DRIED OREGANO
SALT AND FRESHLY GROUND BLACK PEPPER

To serve

250g/9oz/1 CUP GREEK-STYLE YOGURT OR SOUR CREAM
150g/5½oz GLUTEN-FREE CORN CHIPS
115g/4oz CHEDDAR CHEESE, GRATED
CHOPPED FRESH PARSLEY OR CORIANDER (CILANTRO)

Here's a fab, meat-free smoky chipotle and cumin-spiced chilli. Serve with cooling spoonfuls of yogurt, crunchy tortilla chips and grated cheese for a quick midweek supper.

1. Put the chillies in a small bowl, add boiling water to just cover and leave to soak for 5 minutes.

2. Heat the oil in a large saucepan, add the onion and fry gently for 5 minutes, stirring until just beginning to soften and turn golden. Meanwhile, dice 1 of the red peppers, then add to the pan with the beetroot, garlic, cumin and cloves.

3. Stir in the black beans, tomatoes, stock and sugar, then add the bay leaves and oregano. Lift the chillies out of the water, chop and add to the pan together with their seeds and soaking liquid. Season generously with salt and pepper. Bring to the boil, cover and simmer gently for 35–40 minutes, stirring from time to time, until the beetroot is just tender.

4. Spoon into shallow bowls, discarding the bay leaves. Top with spoonfuls of yogurt, corn chips and grated cheese. Finely dice the remaining red pepper and sprinkle over the top, with a little chopped parsley, and serve.

Cook's tip Dried chipotle chillies are becoming more widely available in supermarkets; they can also be bought online. They vary in size, so if you haven't used them before, err on the side of caution as they are fiery! You can always add more at the end of cooking.

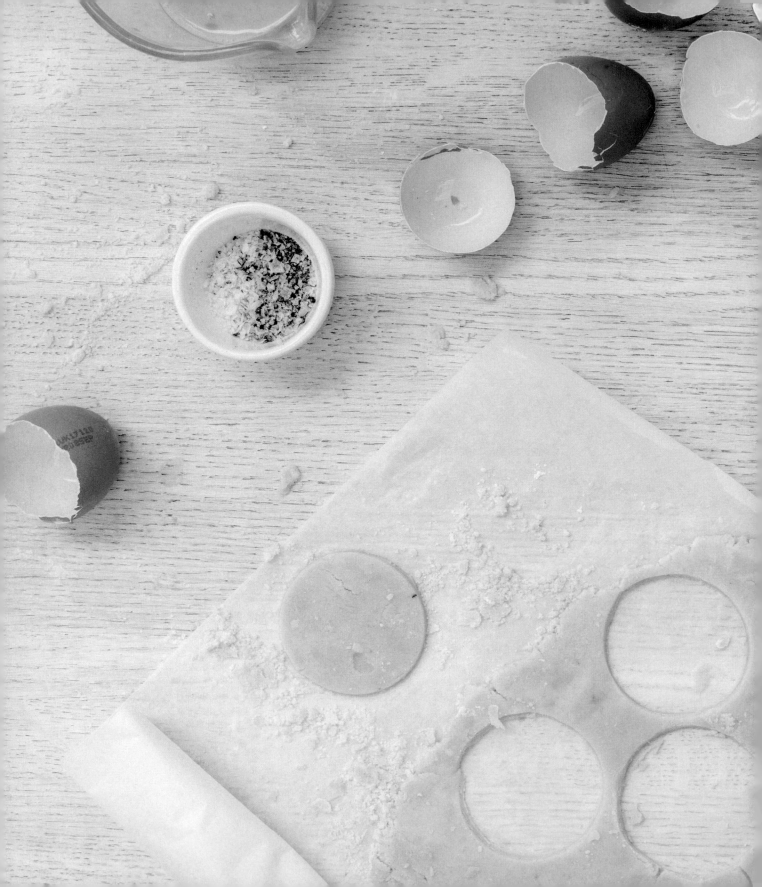

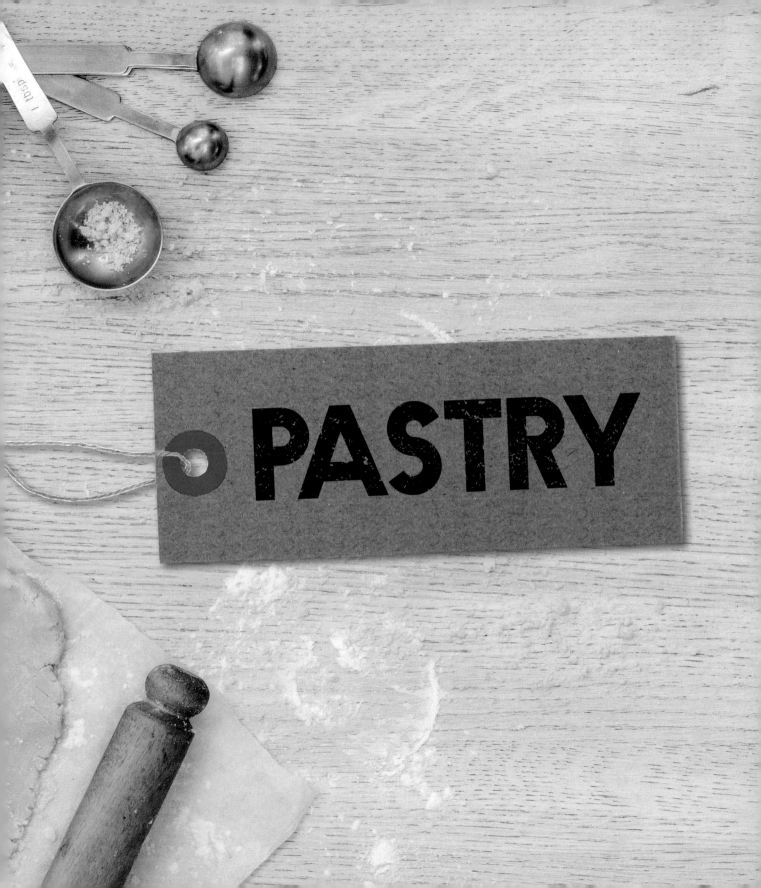

PASTRY

PASTRY

When you think of the vast range of pies and tarts, from golden-topped savoury pies and creamy quiches to luscious fruit tarts, you will be relieved to know that they are most definitely *not* all off the gluten-free menu.

Gluten-free flours produce wonderfully crumbly pastry, but it does need more careful handling than ordinary pastry. Gluten-free pastry is most successful when made with a blend of flours, such as rice and tapioca flours. These have a fine texture and mild flavour and when mixed with butter and egg yolks give a melt-in-the-mouth, almost shortbread-like texture. Polenta adds a pale yellow tinge to pastry, while hemp gives an unusual dark green hue. You might also like to try potato or quinoa flour. Ground almonds, hazelnuts, hemp or sunflower seeds add moistness.

Be adventurous: for savoury pastry why not add a little mustard powder, ground Indian spices or chopped herbs? For sweet pastry replace a little of the soya flour with cocoa or stir in some grated orange or lemon zest, ground cinnamon or vanilla extract.

Traditionally pies and tarts are glazed with beaten egg if they are savoury, milk and sugar if they are sweet, but this is a personal choice. It can also be nice to sprinkle savoury pies with a few salt flakes, thyme or rosemary leaves or a little paprika. For sweet pies, try caster (superfine) or Demerara sugar mixed with a little ground spice or chopped preserved ginger, or dust with sifted icing (confectioners') sugar.

It can be handy to freeze baked but unfilled pastry shells. Cool after baking, then wrap individually in foil and pack into a plastic box so that they don't get damaged. There's no need to defrost them completely before using; take them out of the freezer while you make the filling, then assemble and bake. Rather than tying up all your tart tins in the freezer, you may prefer to make the tarts in disposable freezerproof foil containers.

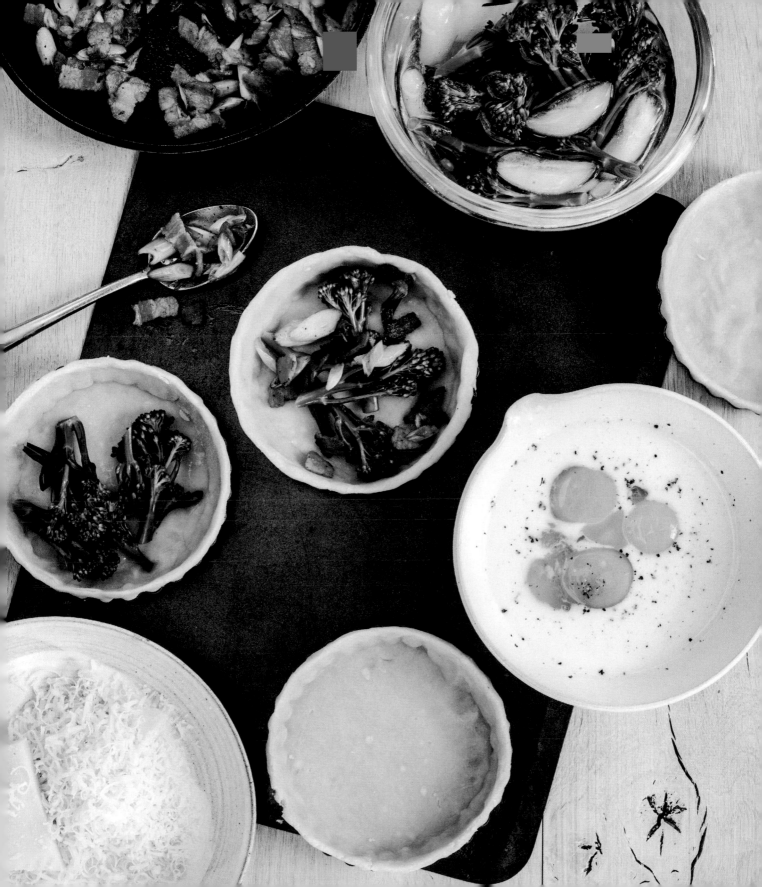

TECHNIQUES

Gluten-free pastry works best with a mix of different gluten-free flours rather than just one type. As there is no gluten in the flour, the dough is much shorter and crumblier than dough made with wheat flour, so it needs to be handled slightly differently.

To help compensate for the lack of gluten, add xanthan gum to the flour mix in a ratio of ½ tsp to 200g/7oz gluten-free flour to aid elasticity. Add fats just as you would when making ordinary pastry. Use butter, white vegetable fat or lard, taken straight from the fridge and diced into small pieces. Rub in with fingertips dipped into the flour or use a food processor or electric mixer.

Add richness to the pastry with egg yolks or whole eggs plus a little cold water, or only water. If mixing by hand, stir in the liquid with a round-bladed knife, then bring the mixture together to make a soft but not sticky dough. If using a food processor it can be harder to tell if the dough is the right consistency, so check at intervals. If the dough is too wet it will be hard when baked. As with any pastry, the less you handle it the lighter it will be.

To avoid cross-contamination with wheat products, knead the pastry lightly on non-stick baking parchment, then roll out between two sheets of parchment. To line a large tart tin, lift off the top sheet of parchment, then invert the pastry into the tin; peel away the second piece of paper once the pastry is in the tin.

Don't worry if the pastry breaks a little, just press any cracks back together or patch with a piece of pastry taken from the trimmings, sticking it in place with a little water or egg yolk. If the pastry looks a little cracked after baking blind (baking without a filling), brush it with beaten egg and put it back in the oven for 5 minutes so that the egg acts as a sealant.

For all tarts, trim the pastry a little above the top of the tins to allow for shrinkage and chill well in the fridge for at least 15 minutes.

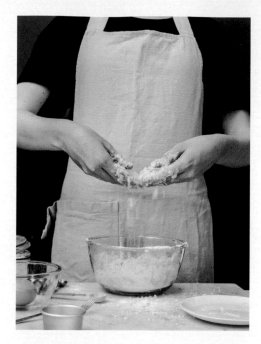

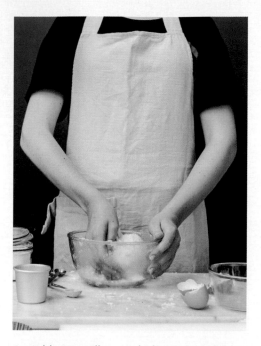

1. Rub in diced butter – or a mix of butter or white vegetable fat or lard – until the mixture looks like fine crumbs.

2. Add egg yolks or whole eggs with a little cold water if needed to mix the pastry to a soft but not sticky dough.

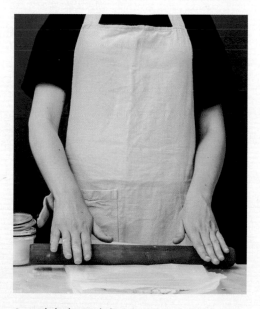

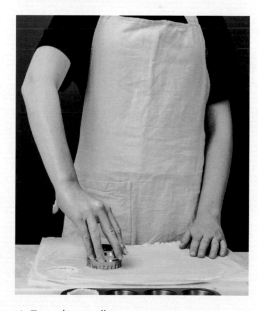

3. Lightly knead the dough, then roll out between two sheets of baking parchment to help prevent it breaking or sticking.

4. To make small tarts or pie tops, stamp out circles with a cutter, then loosen the pastry from the paper with a palette knife.

BEEF EN CROÛTE

SERVES 6
PREP: 1 HOUR, PLUS CHILLING
COOK: 55 MINUTES

800g/1lb 12oz PIECE OF THICK FILLET OF BEEF,
    TIED WITH STRING
SALT AND FRESHLY GROUND BLACK PEPPER
25g/1oz/2 TBSP UNSALTED BUTTER
1 TBSP OLIVE OIL
175g/6oz SHALLOTS, FINELY CHOPPED
300g/10½oz BUTTON MUSHROOMS, FINELY CHOPPED
2 SPRIGS OF THYME, LEAVES ONLY
3 TBSP BRANDY
SMALL BUNCH OF FRESH PARSLEY, CHOPPED
4 CANNED ANCHOVY FILLETS (OPTIONAL),
    DRAINED AND CHOPPED
2 EGG YOLKS
125ml/4fl oz/½ CUP RED WINE
250ml/9fl oz/1 CUP GLUTEN-FREE BEEF STOCK
2 TSP TOMATO PUREE (TOMATO PASTE)

Pastry

175g/6oz/SCANT 1¼ CUPS RICE FLOUR
115g/4oz/SCANT 1 CUP TAPIOCA FLOUR
1 TSP XANTHAN GUM
150g/5½oz/GENEROUS ½ CUP UNSALTED BUTTER, DICED
2 EGGS, BEATEN

Celebrate a special occasion in style with this baked fillet of beef wrapped in a mushroom duxelles and a crumbly buttery pastry, served with a rich red wine sauce. Perfect with potatoes dauphinoise and a simple green vegetable.

1. Sprinkle the beef with salt and pepper. Heat the butter and oil in a frying pan, add the beef and cook over a high heat, turning, until evenly browned, for 6–7 minutes for rare, 9–10 minutes for medium, 12–14 minutes for well done. Lift out of the pan and wrap tightly in baking parchment or foil. Leave to cool to set the shape of the meat.

2. Add the shallots to the pan and cook over a medium heat until softened and just beginning to brown. Add the mushrooms and cook for 3–4 minutes, stirring until any moisture has been driven off. Add the thyme and brandy, heat until the brandy bubbles, then flame with a match. As soon as the flames subside, stir in the parsley and anchovies, if using, and cook for 1 minute. Scoop out two-thirds of the mixture into a bowl, mix with the egg yolks and reserve for the stuffing.

3. Add the wine, stock and tomato purée to the remaining mushrooms in the pan and simmer gently for 5 minutes to make the sauce. Press through a sieve into a small saucepan. Taste and adjust the seasoning.

4. Chill the sauce, seared beef and mushroom stuffing until 1 hour before serving, then take out of the fridge. Preheat the oven to 200°C/400°F/Gas Mark 6.

5. To make the pastry, put the flours, xanthan gum and a little salt and pepper into a bowl or food processor and mix well. Add the butter and rub in until it forms fine crumbs. Gradually mix in about three-quarters of the beaten egg – enough to mix to a soft dough. Knead lightly.

Recipe continues…

Cook's tip Leftover beef tastes delicious cold the next day and is much easier to slice.

GF tip Wheat- and gluten-free pastry are deliciously crumbly and not as easy to cut as pastry made with wheat flour, so don't worry when you come to slice this fab main course.

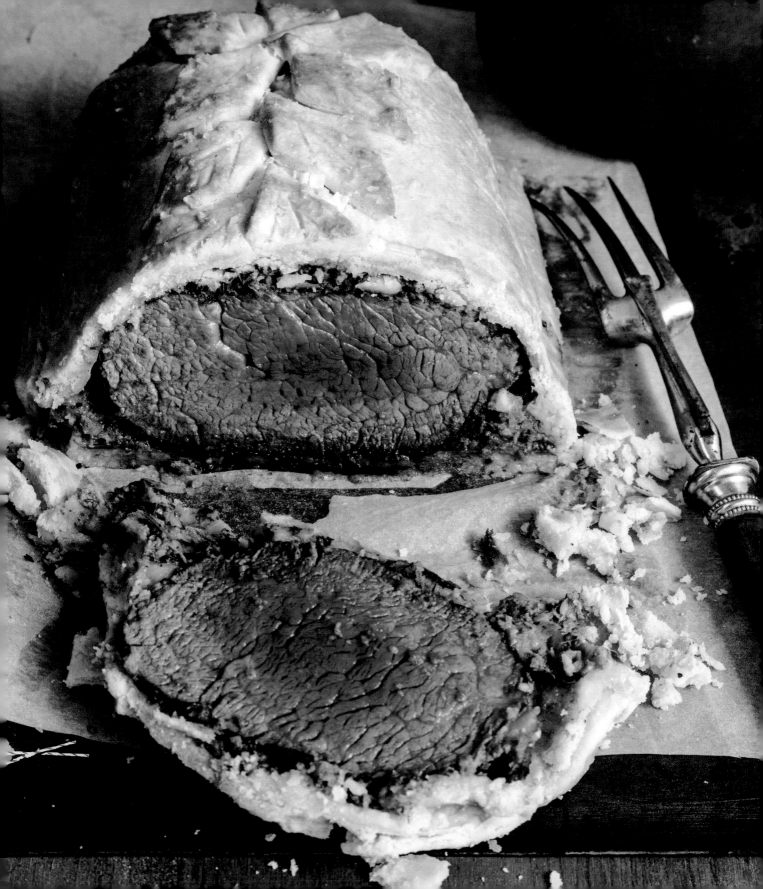

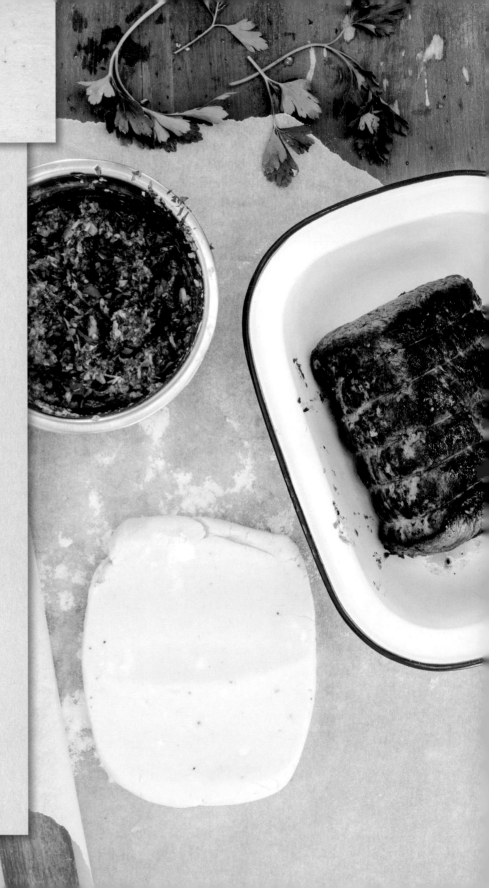

BEEF EN CROÛTE
...CONTINUED

6. Roll out the pastry between 2 sheets of baking parchment to form a square about 33cm/13in. Remove top parchment. Spread half the mushroom stuffing in a strip about the same size as the beef in the centre of the pastry. Unwrap the beef, snip off the string and arrange on top of the mushrooms, adding any juices to the sauce, then spread the remaining mushroom mixture on top of the beef.

7. Brush the edges of the pastry with egg, then bring two sides up and over the long edges of the beef. Press together to seal well. Trim a little of the excess pastry from the ends, then fold up over the beef to make a pastry parcel. Reroll the pastry trimmings and cut out leaf shapes. Brush the parcel with beaten egg, arrange the pastry leaves over the pastry joins and brush with egg.

8. Slide the beef on the parchment on to a baking sheet. Bake for 35 minutes, until the pastry is golden and the beef cooked, brushing the pastry with any remaining egg halfway through cooking.

9. Leave to stand for 10 minutes, then cut into thick slices and serve.

BACON AND BROCCOLI QUICHES

SERVES 4

PREP: 40 MINUTES, PLUS 15–30 MINUTES CHILLING

COOK: 20–25 MINUTES

🍽️⊙🍴

Pastry

150g/5½oz/1 CUP RICE FLOUR,
   PLUS EXTRA FOR DUSTING

55g/2oz/½ CUP FINE POLENTA (CORNMEAL)

1 TSP XANTHAN GUM

SALT AND FRESHLY GROUND BLACK PEPPER

115g/4oz/½ CUP UNSALTED BUTTER, DICED,
   OR HALF BUTTER AND HALF WHITE VEGETABLE FAT

1 EGG, BEATEN

3 TBSP COLD WATER

Filling

85g/3oz TENDERSTEM BROCCOLI (BROCCOLINI),
   CUT INTO BITE-SIZED PIECES

85g/3oz SMOKED STREAKY BACON, CHOPPED,
   OR LARDONS

2 SPRING ONIONS (SCALLIONS), THINLY SLICED

3 EGGS

250ml/9fl oz/1 GENEROUS CUP SEMI-SKIMMED
   (LOW-FAT) MILK

55g/2oz GRUYÈRE CHEESE, FINELY GRATED

These individual quiches are ideal for supper if the family comes home at different times; they're also great in lunchboxes. You will need 4 individual fluted tart tins.

1. To make the pastry, put the rice flour, polenta, xanthan gum and a little salt and pepper into a bowl or food processor and mix well. Add the butter and rub in until it forms fine crumbs. Mix in the egg and as much of the cold water as you need, to make a soft but not sticky dough. Squeeze into a ball.

2. Cut the dough into 4 pieces. Roll out each piece between 2 sheets of baking parchment, lightly dusted with rice flour, to form a circle about 18cm/7in in diameter. Remove the top piece of parchment and invert the pastry into a 13cm/5in fluted tart tin. Remove the other piece of parchment and press the pastry into the bottom and sides of the tin, pressing together any cracks.

3. Using scissors, trim the pastry a little above the top of the tin to allow for shrinkage. Repeat until you have made 4 pastry shells. Put on a baking sheet and chill in the fridge for 15–30 minutes. Preheat the oven to 190°C/375°F/Gas Mark 5.

4. To make the filling, cook the broccoli with some of the tiny leaves in boiling water for 2 minutes. Drain, rinse in iced water and drain again.

5. Dry-fry the bacon over a medium heat until it begins to turn golden. Add the spring onions and cook for a minute or two, until they begin to soften, then remove from the heat. Whisk the eggs, milk, cheese and a little salt and pepper together in a jug.

6. Put the broccoli into the pastry shells, sprinkle with the bacon and spring onions, then pour in the egg custard. Bake for 20–25 minutes, until golden and the pastry is cooked through. Leave to cool for 10 minutes, then serve warm or cool completely.

Recipe continues...

OTHER FLAVOUR COMBOS

• **Roasted red pepper and goat's cheese quiches** – omit the broccoli and bacon. Quarter, deseed and core 1 large red pepper and arrange cut-side downwards in a foil-lined grill pan. Season with salt and pepper and drizzle with 1 tbsp olive oil; grill for 10 minutes or until softened and the skins are charred. Wrap in the foil and leave to cool. When cool, scrape away the pepper skins with a knife, then slice thinly. Divide among the pastry shells, sprinkle with the spring onions, then pour in the egg and milk (don't add the Gruyère) flavoured with 2 tsp finely chopped rosemary leaves. Top with 85g/3oz diced goat's cheese and bake as above.

• **Onion and black olive quiches** – omit the bacon, broccoli and spring onions. Thinly slice 1 large onion and fry gently with 15g/½oz butter and 1 tbsp olive oil for 10 minutes, stirring until softened and just beginning to turn golden. Divide the onion and 55g/2oz pitted and sliced black olives among the pastry shells. Pour in the egg, milk and cheese, then bake as above.

Freezing tip It can be handy to have a supply of dinners for one in the freezer. Fill the raw pastry shells with the blanched broccoli, fried bacon and spring onion, sprinkle the cheese over, then open-freeze until solid. Wrap well in clingfilm (plastic wrap), with the tarts still in the tins. Label and freeze for up to 1 month. To serve, thaw a tart at room temperature for 1 hour. Mix 1 egg with 75ml/2½fl oz/5 tbsp milk and some salt and pepper. Pour this into the tart and bake as above. Freezing without the custard stops the filling from tasting watery when baked.

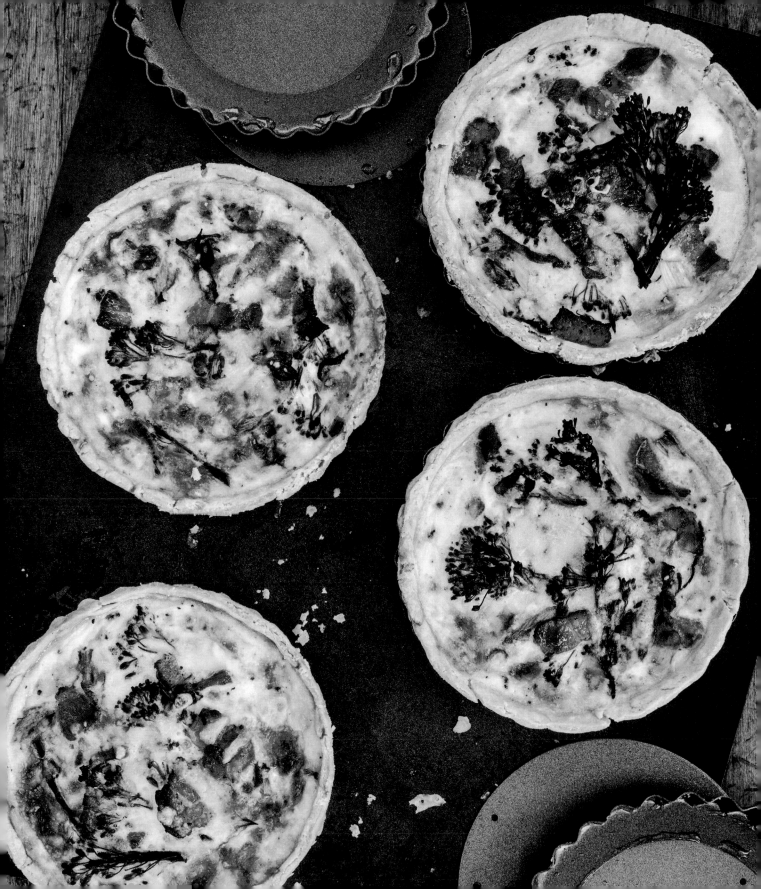

RAISED PORK PIE

SERVES 8–10
PREP: 1 HOUR 15 MINUTES, PLUS OVERNIGHT CHILLING
COOK: 1½ HOURS

Filling

500g/1lb 2oz MINCED (GROUND) PORK
115g/4oz SMOKED BACK BACON, FINELY DICED
200g/7oz SKINLESS, BONELESS CHICKEN BREAST, DICED
4 SPRING ONIONS (SCALLIONS), THINLY SLICED
25g/1oz/3 TBSP DRIED CRANBERRIES
1 TSP BLACK PEPPERCORNS, ROUGHLY CRUSHED
1 TSP FENNEL SEEDS, ROUGHLY CRUSHED
SMALL PIECE OF BLADE MACE, FINELY CRUSHED,
    OR A LARGE PINCH OF GROUND MACE
LARGE PINCH OF GRATED NUTMEG
PINCH OF SALT
115g/4oz READY-TO-EAT DRIED APRICOTS

Hot water crust pastry

175g/6oz/¾ CUP LARD
175ml/6fl oz/¾ CUP SEMI-SKIMMED (LOW-FAT) MILK
115g/4oz/1 CUP BUCKWHEAT FLOUR
115g/4oz/¾ CUP RICE FLOUR
115g/4oz/SCANT 1 CUP TAPIOCA FLOUR
1 TSP XANTHAN GUM
SALT AND FRESHLY GROUND BLACK PEPPER
1 EGG, BEATEN, TO GLAZE

Jelly

2 SHEETS OF LEAF GELATINE
150ml/5fl oz/⅔ CUP MEDIUM OR DRY CIDER,
    OR GLUTEN-FREE CHICKEN STOCK
2 TBSP FINELY CHOPPED FRESH PARSLEY

This classic British pie is best made a day ahead and well chilled. It's perfect for picnics or as part of a cold buffet with other cold meats, pickles and salad.

1. Preheat the oven to 180°C/350°F/Gas Mark 4. To make the filling, put all the ingredients except the apricots into a large bowl and mix together with a fork.

2. To make the pastry, put the lard and milk in a saucepan and heat gently until the lard has completely melted. In a bowl, mix together the flours, xanthan gum, salt and pepper. Bring the milk mixture just to the boil, remove from the heat, add the flour mixture and keep stirring to form a rough ball. Leave to cool for 5 minutes.

3. Cut off one-quarter of the dough and set aside, wrapped in foil. Tip the rest of the dough into a deep 18cm/7in loose-bottomed cake tin (no need to grease it). Working quickly, press the hot pastry over the bottom and up the sides of the tin with your knuckles and fingertips in an even layer. Trim the pastry level with the top of the tin and reserve the trimmings.

4. Spoon half the pork mixture into the pastry-lined tin and press down with the back of a fork. Arrange the apricots in a layer on top, then cover with the remaining pork mixture.

5. Combine the pastry trimmings with the reserved pastry, then roll out between 2 sheets of baking parchment to form a rough circle a little larger than the top of the tin. Brush the pastry edges in the tin with beaten egg, then press the pastry lid in place and squeeze the top edges together to seal well. Trim off the excess pastry and reserve.

6. Crimp the top edge of the pie and brush with beaten egg. Reroll the pastry trimmings between 2 sheets of parchment and cut out leaf shapes. Arrange these on the top of the pie and glaze the leaves with egg. Make a small hole in the centre of the pie for the steam to escape.

7. Bake for 1½ hours; after 30–45 minutes, brush once more

Recipe continues...

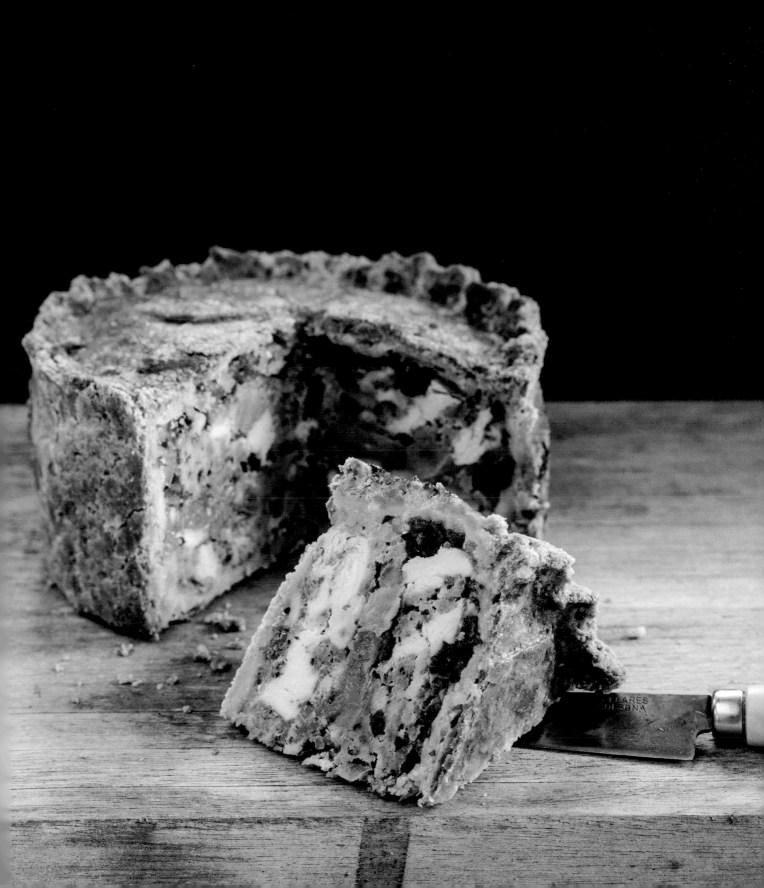

RAISED PORK PIE
...CONTINUED

with egg glaze; after 1 hour, cover with foil to stop the top from browning too much. Remove from the oven and leave to cool overnight.

8. To fill with jelly, put the gelatine in a shallow dish, add enough cold water to cover and leave for 5 minutes. Bring the cider just to the boil in a saucepan, then remove from the heat. Drain the gelatine sheets, add to the cider and stir until dissolved. Season with salt and pepper and stir in the parsley. Leave to cool. Slightly enlarge the hole in the top of the pie and pour in the cooled jelly through a small funnel. Leave for 3–4 hours or overnight for the jelly to set.

9. Run a palette knife around the sides of the tin to loosen the pie, remove the tin and put the pie on a chopping board. Cut into wedges and serve with pickles and salad. Wrap any leftovers in foil and store in the fridge for 2–3 days.

Cook's tips

Most of the pastry is pressed over the bottom and sides of the tin, and unlike shortcrust pastry you don't need to worry about having a light touch. Mould the pastry while hot, or as hot as your hands can stand – it's more pliable that way. Try to keep the pastry an even thickness and make sure there are no holes or the meat juices can run out during cooking and make the pie stick to the tin.

If you are not a fan of jelly, or are short of time, then simply leave out step 8.

CHICKEN POT PIES

This is a useful dish for when you're juggling chores, as the chicken simmers while you get on with something else. You can make the pies and leave them in the fridge until you're ready to bake them.

SERVES 6

PREP: 1 HOUR, PLUS COOLING

COOK: 2 HOURS FOR THE CHICKEN AND SAUCE;
   30–35 MINUTES TO BAKE THE PIES

1 CHICKEN, WEIGHING ABOUT 1.3kg/3lb,
   RINSED INSIDE AND OUT

1 ONION, QUARTERED

2 CARROTS, THICKLY SLICED

SALT AND FRESHLY GROUND BLACK PEPPER

1.5 LITRES/2½ PINTS/7 CUPS COLD WATER

1 TBSP OLIVE OIL

2 SMALL LEEKS, THICKLY SLICED

150g/5½oz BUTTON MUSHROOMS, SLICED

3 SPRIGS OF FRESH TARRAGON, LEAVES FINELY CHOPPED

2 TBSP GLUTEN-FREE CORNFLOUR (CORNSTARCH)

Pastry

175g/6oz/SCANT 1¼ CUPS RICE FLOUR

115g/4oz/SCANT 1 CUP TAPIOCA FLOUR

1 TSP XANTHAN GUM

150g/5½oz/GENEROUS ½ CUP UNSALTED BUTTER,
   OR HALF BUTTER AND HALF WHITE VEGETABLE FAT, DICED

2 EGGS, BEATEN

SEA SALT FLAKES, TO FINISH (OPTIONAL)

1. Put the chicken breast-side down into a saucepan in which it fits snugly. Add the onion, carrots and plenty of salt and pepper, then pour in enough of the cold water to just cover the chicken. Bring to the boil, then reduce the heat, cover and simmer for 1 hour 20 minutes, until just tender and the juices run clear when the chicken is pierced through the thickest part of the leg.

2. Lift the chicken out onto a plate, wrap in foil and leave to cool. Simmer the stock, uncovered, for about 30 minutes to reduce it down to about 600ml/20fl oz/2½ cups.

3. Heat the oil in a deep frying pan, add the leeks and mushrooms and fry gently for about 5 minutes, stirring until the mushrooms are just beginning to turn golden. Add the tarragon, then strain the stock and add to the pan. Mix the cornflour with a little water to make a smooth paste, stir into the pan and simmer, stirring until the sauce has thickened. Remove from the heat and leave to cool. Put the chicken and sauce in the fridge until ready to assemble the pies.

4. Take the meat off the chicken bones, discarding the skin, and cut the meat into bite-sized pieces. Divide among 6 individual 200–250ml/7–9fl oz/approx. 1 cup pie dishes or metal pudding moulds, spoon the tarragon sauce over the top, then put the dishes on a baking sheet. Preheat the oven to 190°C/375°F/Gas Mark 5.

5. To make the pastry, put the flours, xanthan gum and a pinch of salt into a bowl or food processor and mix well. Add the fats and rub in until it forms fine crumbs. Add three-quarters of

Recipe continues...

CHICKEN POT PIE
...CONTINUED

the egg and mix to a smooth, soft dough, adding about 1 tbsp cold water if needed. Knead lightly, then cut into 6 pieces.

6. Roll out each piece of pastry between 2 sheets of baking parchment, then use a pastry cutter to cut out a neat circle to fit the top of the pie dish. Wet the rim of the dish, press the pastry in place and crimp the edge. Repeat to make 6 pies. Reroll the pastry trimmings and cut out leaves or other shapes. Stick onto the pie tops, using a little of the beaten egg, then use the remaining egg to glaze the pie tops. Sprinkle with salt flakes if liked.

7. Bake for 30–35 minutes, until the pastry is golden brown and the filling is bubbling. Serve with steamed green vegetables.

Cook's tip When poaching the chicken, you could replace some of the water with white wine or dry cider or a few tablespoons of dry sherry.

Freezing tip You might like to eat two pies now and freeze four for another night. Make the pies as in step 6 but do not sprinkle with salt flakes. Open-freeze on a tray until firm. Wrap in clingfilm (plastic wrap), pack in a large plastic box and label. Thaw overnight in the fridge. Remove the clingfilm and bake as in step 7.

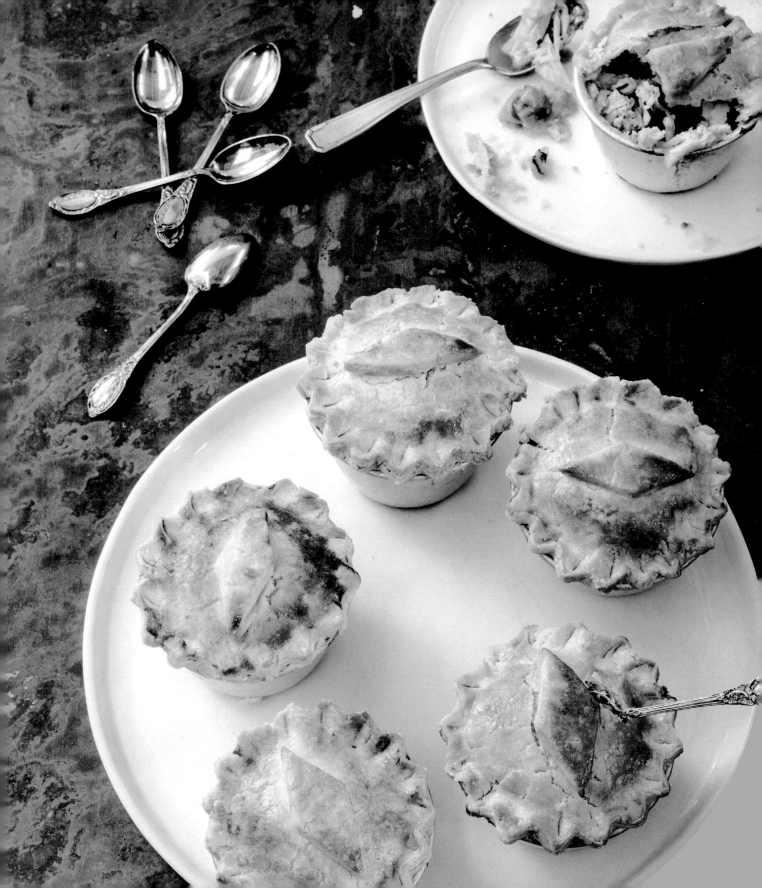

INDIVIDUAL FISH PIES

SERVES 4

PREP: 30 MINUTES, PLUS COOLING

COOK: 40 MINUTES

25g/1oz/2 TBSP UNSALTED BUTTER
1 TBSP SUNFLOWER OIL
55g/2oz SMOKED STREAKY BACON, DICED
1 ONION, CHOPPED
300g/10½oz POTATOES, PEELED AND DICED
1 FENNEL BULB, DICED
450ml/16fl oz/2 CUPS GLUTEN-FREE FISH STOCK
1 BAY LEAF
350g/12oz MONKFISH OR OTHER FIRM WHITE FISH
    FILLETS, SKINNED AND SLICED
350g/12oz SALMON FILLET, SKINNED AND CUBED
SALT AND FRESHLY GROUND BLACK PEPPER
6 TBSP FULL-FAT CRÈME FRAÎCHE

Pastry

175g/6oz/SCANT 1¼ CUPS RICE FLOUR
115g/4oz/SCANT 2 CUPS POTATO FLOUR
½ TSP XANTHAN GUM
150g/5½oz/GENEROUS ½ CUP UNSALTED BUTTER, DICED
SMALL BUNCH OF FRESH PARSLEY, FINELY CHOPPED
SMALL BUNCH OF FRESH CHIVES, FINELY CHOPPED
2 EGGS

Break through the green speckled herb pastry to an American-style fish chowder flavoured with smoked bacon, fennel and crème fraîche. The potatoes thicken the filling, so there is no need to make a separate sauce.

1. Heat the butter and oil in a frying pan, add the bacon and onion and cook over a medium heat for 5 minutes, stirring, until the bacon and onion are just beginning to colour. Mix in the potatoes and fennel, cover and cook gently for 5 minutes.

2. Add the stock, bay leaf and fish and season with a little salt and pepper. Bring to the boil, then cover and simmer gently for 5 minutes, until the fish is only just cooked. Leave to cool. Spoon into 4 individual 450ml/16fl oz/2 cup pie dishes and stir in the crème fraîche.

3. Preheat the oven to 190°C/375°F/Gas Mark 5. To make the pastry, put the flours, xanthan gum and some salt and pepper into a bowl or food processor and mix well. Add the butter and rub in until it forms fine crumbs. Add the chopped herbs and 1 egg; beat the second egg in a separate bowl. Mix the dough until it forms a soft ball, adding a little of the beaten egg if needed.

4. Knead the dough very lightly, then cut into 4 pieces. Roll out each piece between 2 sheets of baking parchment until a little larger than the top of a pie dish. Brush the dish with a little of the beaten egg, add the pastry lid, press to the edge of the dish and trim off any excess pastry. Repeat to make 4 pies. Press a fork onto the edges of the pies to decorate. Brush the pastry with a little of the remaining egg to glaze.

5. Bake for about 25 minutes, until the pastry is golden brown and the filling is bubbling. Serve with steamed green beans.

Cook's tip You can leave out the bacon if you prefer.

Freezing tip You might like to eat two pies now and freeze two for another night. Make the pies up to the end of step 4 and open-freeze until the pastry is hard. Wrap in foil and label. Thaw overnight in the fridge. Remove the foil and bake as above.

MEDITERRANEAN PICNIC PIES

MAKES 6
PREP: 50 MINUTES
COOK: 30 MINUTES, PLUS COOLING

3 MIXED PEPPERS (RED, ORANGE, YELLOW OR GREEN),
    QUARTERED, CORED AND DESEEDED
2 COURGETTES (ZUCCHINI), CUT INTO THICK SLICES
8 SHALLOTS, HALVED
115g/4oz CHERRY TOMATOES
4 GARLIC CLOVES, SEPARATED BUT NOT PEELED
2 TBSP OLIVE OIL
SALT AND FRESHLY GROUND BLACK PEPPER
1 TBSP BALSAMIC VINEGAR

Pastry

150g/5½oz/1¼ CUPS COARSE POLENTA (CORNMEAL)
55g/2oz/½ CUP TAPIOCA FLOUR, PLUS EXTRA FOR
    DUSTING
½ TSP XANTHAN GUM
115g/4oz/½ CUP UNSALTED BUTTER, DICED
55g/2oz PARMESAN CHEESE, GRATED,
    PLUS EXTRA FOR SPRINKLING
1 EGG, PLUS 1 EGG, BEATEN, TO GLAZE

Cook's tip If you don't have any individual tart tins, make pasties instead. Spoon some of the vegetable filling onto each rolled-out circle of pastry, then brush the edges of the pastry with egg, fold in half, and press the edges together to make a pasty.

Coarse polenta mixed with grated Parmesan makes an unusual pastry that works well with the grilled vegetables and tastes just as good hot or cold. If taking on a picnic, transport them in their tins, wrapped in foil.

1. Preheat the grill (broiler) and line the grill pan with foil. Place the peppers on the grill pan, cut-side down, in a single layer, then add the courgettes in a single layer, and tuck the shallots, tomatoes and garlic among the peppers. Drizzle with the oil and sprinkle with salt and pepper. Grill for 10–15 minutes, until the pepper skins have blackened, the shallots and courgettes are tender and the tomatoes softened.

2. Wrap the foil around the vegetables and leave to cool for 5 minutes so that the pepper skins loosen.

3. Open out the foil, peel away the pepper skins and garlic skins. Dice the peppers, shallots and courgettes and finely chop the garlic. Mix the vegetables with the pan juices and balsamic vinegar and leave to cool. Preheat the oven to 190°C/375°F/ Gas Mark 5.

4. To make the pastry, put the polenta, tapioca flour and xanthan gum into a bowl or food processor and mix well. Add the butter and rub in until it forms fine crumbs. Stir in the grated Parmesan, add 1 egg and mix in 1–2 tsp cold water – just enough to make a soft but not sticky dough. Squeeze into a ball.

5. Cut the dough into 6 pieces. Roll out one piece between 2 sheets of baking parchment, lightly dusted with tapioca flour, to form a rough circle about 18cm/7in in diameter. Remove the top piece of parchment and gently invert the pastry into a 10cm/4in straight-sided shallow tart tin or Yorkshire pudding tin; peel off the other piece of parchment, then pleat and fold the pastry so that it stands above the top of the tin. Spoon in one sixth of the vegetable mixture, then fold the pastry down over the filling, leaving the centre uncovered. Repeat to make 6 pies.

6. Brush the tops with a little beaten egg and sprinkle with a little grated Parmesan. Bake for 18–20 minutes, until golden brown. Serve warm or leave until cold, then wrap in foil to add to a lunchbox or picnic basket.

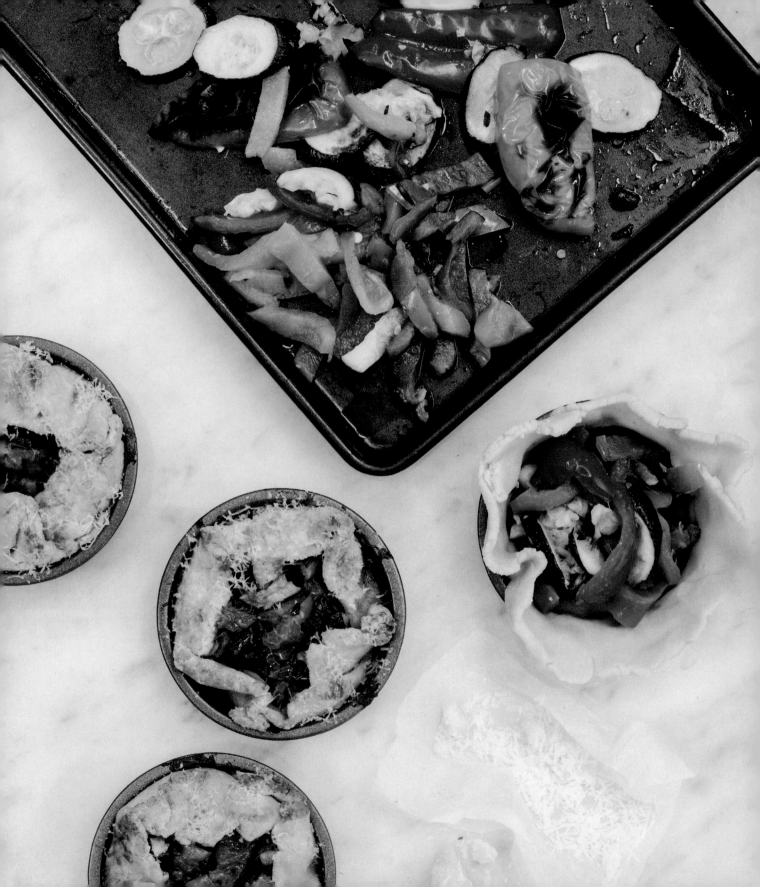

FILLING VARIATIONS

- **Creamy spinach** – wash 200g/7oz spinach, drain well, then cook in a large pan for 2–3 minutes with just the water clinging to the leaves, until just wilted. Cool, then chop. Beat 200g/7oz full-fat cream cheese with 2 eggs, 2 finely chopped garlic cloves, a pinch of grated nutmeg and salt and freshly ground black pepper. Stir in the spinach. Fill the pies as in step 5 and bake.

- **Cauliflower cheese** – cut 1 small cauliflower into small florets and steam for 8–10 minutes, until just tender. Melt 25g/1oz/2 tbsp unsalted butter in a saucepan, stir in 40g/1½oz/3 tbsp rice flour, then gradually mix in 300ml/10fl oz/1¼ cups milk and bring to the boil, stirring, until thickened and smooth. Stir in 2 tsp wholegrain mustard, 115g/4oz grated mature Cheddar cheese and salt and freshly ground black pepper. Cool for 15 minutes, then mix in 1 beaten egg and the cauliflower. Fill the pies as in step 5 and bake.

- **Garlic mushroom** – fry 1 finely chopped onion in 1 tbsp olive oil for 5 minutes, stirring, until softened. Mix in 2 finely chopped garlic cloves and 250g/9oz small whole button mushrooms and fry for 2 minutes. Mix in a 400g can chopped tomatoes, 1 tbsp tomato purée (tomato paste), salt and freshly ground black pepper. Cook, uncovered, over a medium heat for 5 minutes, until the sauce has thickened. Stir in a small handful of torn basil and leave to cool. Fill the pies as in step 5 and bake.

GF tip Gluten-free pastry is very fragile, so don't worry too much if the pastry cracks, just press it together where you can – it's all part of the rustic charm.

PECORINO CHEESE STRAWS

MAKES 30
PREP: 25 MINUTES
COOK: 10 MINUTES

55g/2oz/½ CUP FINE POLENTA (CORNMEAL)
85g/3oz/GENEROUS ½ CUP RICE FLOUR,
  PLUS EXTRA FOR DUSTING
85g/3oz/6 TBSP UNSALTED BUTTER, DICED
1 TSP GLUTEN-FREE MUSTARD POWDER,
  SUCH AS COLMAN'S
SALT AND FRESHLY GROUND BLACK PEPPER
2 TSP ROUGHLY CHOPPED FRESH THYME LEAVES
70g/2½oz PECORINO CHEESE, FINELY GRATED
2 EGGS

Perfect with a chilled glass of wine, or as a treat added to work or school lunchboxes.

1. Preheat the oven to 180°C/350°F/Gas Mark 4. Put the polenta and flour into a mixing bowl, then rub in the butter until it forms fine crumbs.

2. Stir in the mustard, salt and pepper, half the thyme and 55g/2oz of the cheese. In a small bowl, beat 1 egg with a fork, add to the flour mixture, then beat the second egg and add 1 tbsp or just enough to make a soft dough. Squeeze into a ball.

3. Roll out the dough between 2 sheets of baking parchment, lightly dusted with rice flour, to form a rough 25cm/10in square. Peel off the top piece of parchment, cut the square in half, then cut each half into thin strips about 1cm/½in wide. Brush lightly with some of the remaining beaten egg.

4. Lift the parchment onto a large baking sheet and separate the strips slightly. Sprinkle with the remaining thyme leaves and cheese, and a little coarsely crushed black pepper, if liked.

5. Bake for about 10 minutes, until golden brown. Leave to cool on the baking parchment. Store any leftovers in an airtight plastic container for 2–3 days.

Cook's tip If serving these to children, don't sprinkle the tops with thyme and black pepper, but add a sprinkling of sesame seeds instead. Pecorino can be substitued for Parmesan.

GF tip Gluten-free pastry can be very crumbly to roll out, but rolling between 2 sheets of baking parchment makes it quick and simple, and there's no need to prepare a baking sheet – just transfer the parchment to the baking sheet.

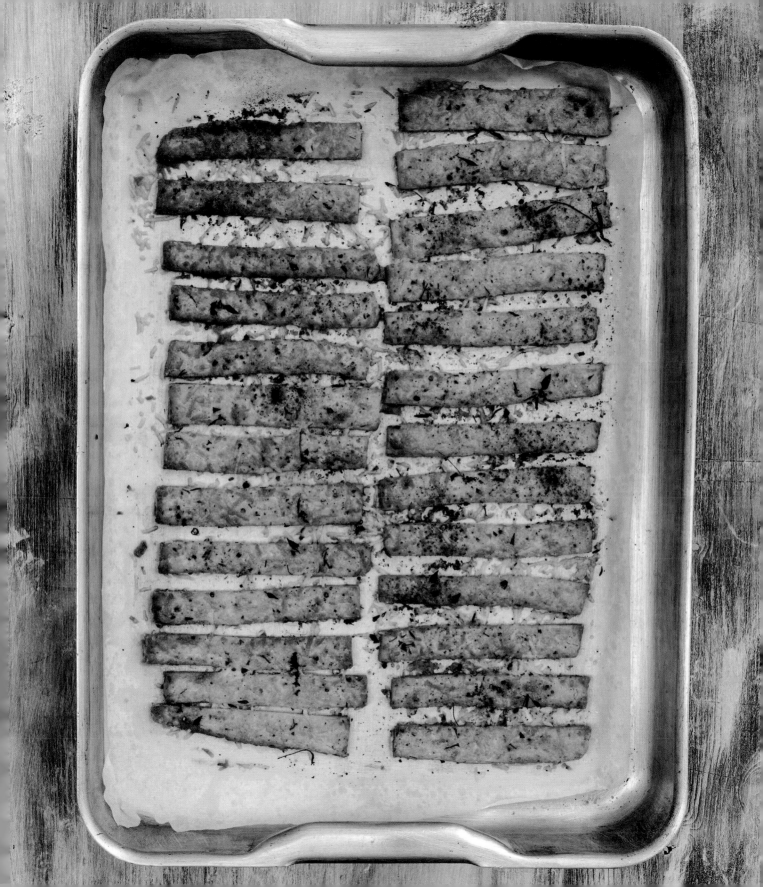

HAZELNUT AND LEEK TART

SERVES 6–8

PREP: 10 MINUTES, PLUS 15–30 MINUTES CHILLING

COOK: 45–60 MINUTES

Pastry

55g/2oz/SCANT ½ CUP HAZELNUTS

55g/2oz/½ CUP HEMP FLOUR

115g/4oz/¾ CUP RICE FLOUR,
    PLUS EXTRA FOR DUSTING

½ TSP XANTHAN GUM

SALT AND FRESHLY GROUND BLACK PEPPER

115g/4oz/½ CUP UNSALTED BUTTER, DICED

2 EGG YOLKS

3 TSP COLD WATER

Filling

25g/1oz/2 TBSP UNSALTED BUTTER

2 TRIMMED LEEKS, ABOUT 300G/10½OZ, THINLY SLICED

150ml/5fl oz/⅔ CUP DOUBLE (HEAVY) CREAM

150ml/5fl oz/⅔ CUP SEMI-SKIMMED (LOW-FAT) MILK

4 EGGS

1 TBSP FINELY CHOPPED FRESH TARRAGON

250g/9oz CAMEMBERT, CUT INTO 10–12 WEDGES

This is no ordinary quiche. Hemp flour is the most amazing dark greeny-brown colour, so it makes a distinctive-looking pastry with a slightly nutty flavour.

1. To make the pastry, put the hazelnuts in a small pan over a medium heat until golden brown, shaking the pan so that they colour evenly. Leave to cool, then chop very finely or blitz in a food processor.

2. Put the nuts, flours, xanthan gum and a little salt and pepper into a bowl or food processor and mix well. Add the butter and rub in until it forms fine crumbs. Mix in the egg yolks and as much of the cold water as you need, to make a soft but not sticky dough. Squeeze into a ball.

3. Dust your fingers with rice flour, then press the pastry over the bottom and up the sides of a 25cm/10in loose-bottomed fluted tart tin in a thin, even layer; the pastry should stand a little above the top of the tin. Neaten the top edge with scissors, if necessary. Prick the bottom with a fork, then chill for 15–30 minutes. Preheat the oven to 190°C/375°F/Gas Mark 5.

4. Line the pastry shell with baking parchment and dried beans and bake for 10 minutes. Remove the paper and beans and cook for 5–10 minutes, until the pastry is crisp.

5. To make the filling, heat the butter in a frying pan, add the leeks and cook for a few minutes, stirring, until just softened. In a bowl, beat together the cream, milk and eggs with the tarragon and a generous amount of salt and pepper.

6. Spoon the leeks into the pastry, pour in the tarragon custard, then arrange the Camembert on top. Bake for 30–40 minutes, until the top is golden and the custard set. Leave to cool for 10 minutes, then cut into wedges to serve.

Cook's tips

Add some medium-sized baking potatoes to the oven while the pastry chills, and by the time the tart is cooked the potatoes will be ready. Toss a salad with some balsamic vinegar for a great supper.

Any leftover tart can be packed into lunchboxes the next day.

Freezing tip Blind-bake the pastry shell as in step 4 and leave to cool in the tin. Wrap in clingfilm, still in the tin, label and freeze for up to 3 months. Thaw for 1 hour at room temperature, then fill and bake.

DOUBLE CRUST BLACKBERRY AND APPLE PIE

SERVES 6
PREP: 35 MINUTES
COOK: 30–35 MINUTES

Filling

1kg/2lb 4oz COOKING APPLES, CORED,
    PEELED AND SLICED
150g/5½oz/1 CUP BLACKBERRIES
85g/3oz/SCANT ½ CUP CASTER (SUPERFINE) SUGAR
2 TBSP GROUND ALMONDS
1 TSP GROUND CINNAMON

Pastry

175g/6oz/SCANT 1¼ CUPS RICE FLOUR
115g/4oz/SCANT 1 CUP TAPIOCA FLOUR
55g/2oz/7 PACKED LEVEL TBSP SOYA FLOUR
55g/2oz/¼ CUP CASTER (SUPERFINE) SUGAR,
    PLUS EXTRA FOR SPRINKLING
1 TSP GROUND CINNAMON
1 TSP XANTHAN GUM
175g/6oz/¾ CUP UNSALTED BUTTER, DICED
2 EGGS, PLUS 1 EGG YOLK
3 TBSP COLD WATER

Cook's tip To avoid a soggy-bottomed pie always use a metal pie plate: this will conduct heat well and help to crisp up the pastry. The ground almonds help to absorb any excess apple juice which could also make the bottom of the pie go soft.

A comforting family pudding, delicious served warm with cream, gluten-free custard or a spoonful of good-quality vanilla ice cream.

1. Preheat the oven to 190°C/375°F/Gas Mark 5. Mix all the filling ingredients together in a bowl.

2. To make the pastry, put the flours, sugar, cinnamon and xanthan gum into a bowl or food processor and mix well. Add the butter and rub in until it forms fine crumbs.

3. Separate 1 egg, reserve the white for glazing, and add the yolk, the extra yolk and the whole egg to the flours. Add enough of the cold water to make a soft but not sticky dough.

4. Reserve one-third of the dough for the top; lightly knead and roll out the rest between 2 large sheets of baking parchment until large enough to line a 25cm/10in diameter metal pie dish (4cm/1½in deep). Peel off the top layer of parchment, then invert the pastry into the dish and peel off the second piece of parchment. Press the pastry into the dish and trim off any excess.

5. Spoon the apple mixture into the pie dish. Roll out the reserved pastry together with any trimmings between parchment until about 25cm/10in long. Cut 2.5cm/1in wide strips and arrange over the pie in a lattice, sticking the ends in place with the reserved egg white. Reroll any trimmings until the top is covered with a lattice of pastry.

6. Brush the pastry with egg white, sprinkle with a little sugar and bake for 30–35 minutes, until the pastry is golden brown and the apples are tender. Check after 20 minutes and cover the top loosely with foil if the pastry seems to be browning too quickly. Serve warm, cut into wedges.

Recipe continues…

FILLING VARIATIONS

• **Plum and blueberry** – replace the apples with 750g/1lb 10oz sliced and stoned plums.

• **Cranberry, apple and orange** – replace with blackberries with 150g/5½oz defrosted frozen cranberries, and replace the cinnamon with the grated zest of 1 orange and 1 tsp ground mixed spice (pumpkin pie spice).

• **Peach and raspberry** – replace the apples with 750g/1lb 10oz sliced and stoned ripe peaches (no need to peel), and the blackberries with 150g/5½oz raspberries. Replace with cinnamon with the grated zest of 1 unwaxed lemon. Reduce the caster sugar to 55g/2oz.

• **Christmas pear and mincemeat** – replace with apples with the same weight of peeled, cored and sliced pears mixed with the grated zest of ½ large orange and ½ unwaxed lemon. Omit the blackberries, sugar, almonds and cinnamon. Spoon into the pie dish, then spoon over 150g/5½oz gluten-free mincemeat.

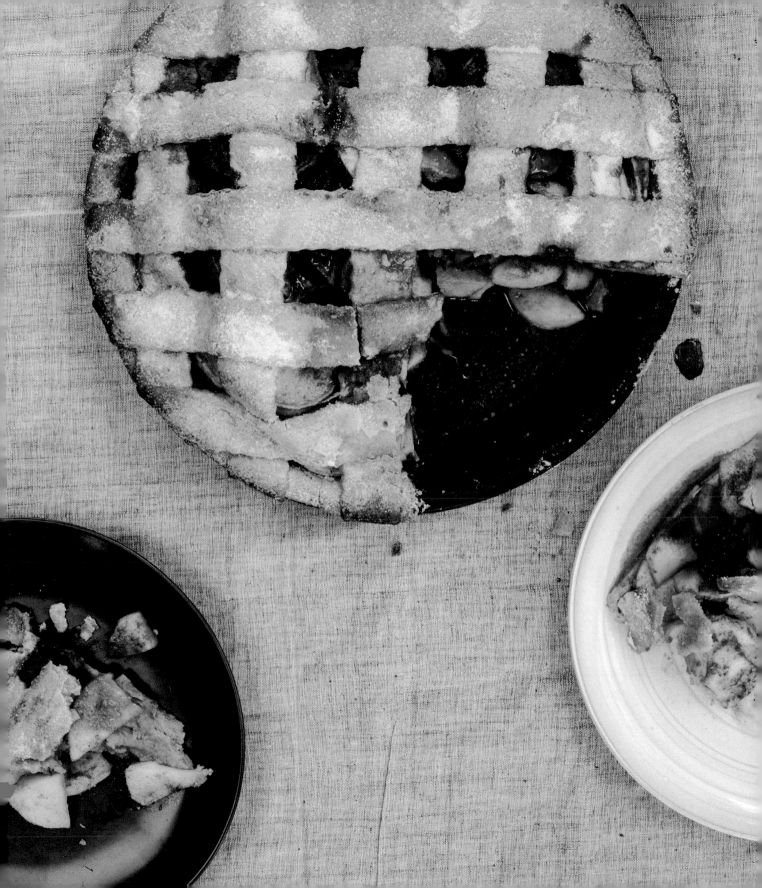

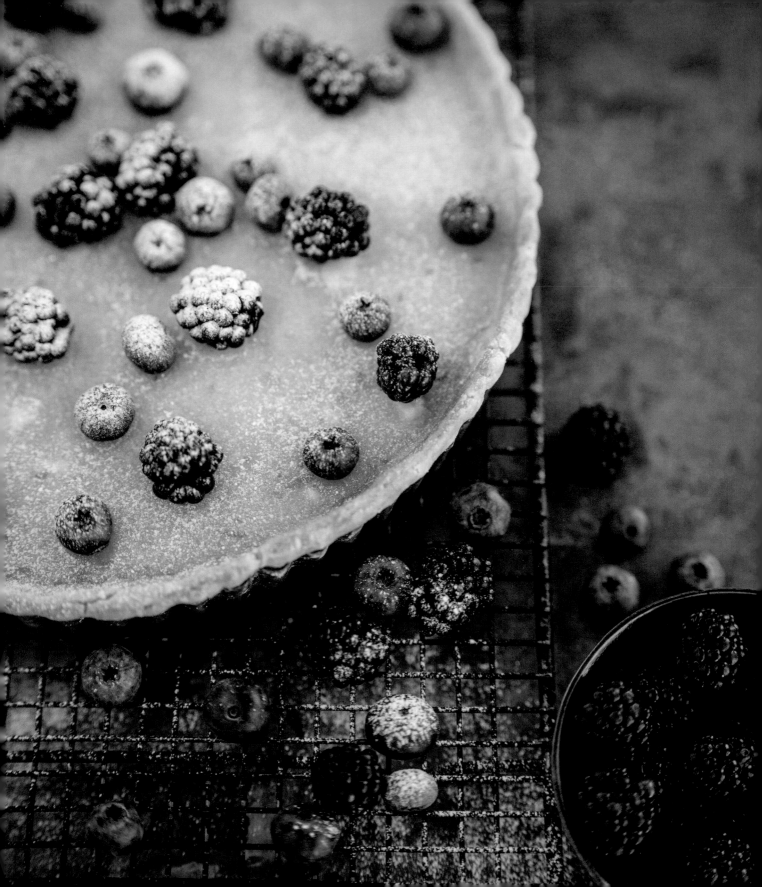

LEMON
AND LIME TART

SERVES 8

PREP: 35 MINUTES, PLUS 15–30 MINUTES CHILLING

COOK: 40–50 MINUTES

Almond pastry

115g/4oz/¾ CUP RICE FLOUR,
    PLUS EXTRA FOR DUSTING
55g/2oz/½ CUP TAPIOCA FLOUR
½ TSP XANTHAN GUM
55g/2oz/½ CUP GROUND ALMONDS
2 TBSP CASTER (SUPERFINE) SUGAR
115g/4oz/½ CUP UNSALTED BUTTER, DICED
1 EGG
1–2 TSP COLD WATER

Filling

GRATED ZEST AND JUICE OF 2 UNWAXED LEMONS
GRATED ZEST AND JUICE OF 2 LIMES
225g/8oz/GENEROUS 1 CUP CASTER (SUPERFINE) SUGAR
150g/5½oz/GENEROUS ½ CUP UNSALTED BUTTER, DICED
4 EGGS
2 EGG YOLKS
GLUTEN-FREE ICING (CONFECTIONERS') SUGAR,
    FOR DUSTING
BLACKBERRIES AND BLUEBERRIES, TO SERVE

This can be made the night before and kept chilled in the fridge (or frozen; thaw overnight in the fridge): allow to come to room temperature for 30 minutes or so before serving. Delicious with fresh berries and a spoonful of crème fraîche.

1. To make the pastry, put the flours, xanthan gum, almonds and sugar into a bowl or food processor and mix well. Add the butter and rub in until it forms fine crumbs. Stir in the egg and mix in the cold water, if needed, to make a soft but not sticky dough. Squeeze into a ball.

2. Dust your fingers with rice flour and press the dough over the bottom and up the sides of a 25cm/10in loose-bottomed fluted tart tin, making a thin even layer; the pastry should stand a little above the top of the tin. Neaten the edge with scissors if necessary. Prick the bottom with a fork, then chill in the fridge for 15–30 minutes.

3. Preheat the oven to 190°C/375°F/Gas Mark 5. Line the pastry with baking parchment and a layer of dried beans and bake for 10 minutes. Carefully remove the paper and beans and bake for an additional 5–8 minutes, until the bottom of the pastry is cooked through.

4. Meanwhile, make the filling: put the lemon and lime zest and juice in a saucepan, add the sugar and butter and cook over a gentle heat, stirring, until the butter has melted and the sugar dissolved. Leave to cool for 10 minutes, then gradually stir in the eggs and egg yolks, until smooth.

5. Pour the filling into the pastry shell. Reduce the oven to 140°C/275°F/Gas Mark 1 and cook for 30–40 minutes, or until the filling is set. Leave to cool. Remove the tart from the tin and transfer to a serving plate. To serve, dust with a little sifted icing sugar and scatter over a few berries.

GF tip Gluten-free pastry is very delicate and crumbly, so if you find that the pastry has cracked after baking blind you can stick the cracks together by brushing with a little beaten egg and baking for another 2 minutes to set the egg 'glue'.

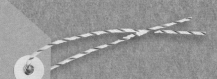

MILE HIGH
STRAWBERRY TARTS

MAKES 6
PREP: 1 HOUR 15 MINUTES, PLUS 30 MINUTES CHILLING
COOK: 15 MINUTES

Pastry shells

115g/4oz/¾ CUP RICE FLOUR,
    PLUS EXTRA FOR DUSTING
55g/2oz/½ CUP TAPIOCA FLOUR
½ TSP XANTHAN GUM
1½ TBSP UNSWEETENED COCOA POWDER
25g/1oz/2 TBSP CASTER (SUPERFINE) SUGAR
115g/4oz/½ CUP UNSALTED BUTTER, DICED
2 EGG YOLKS
115g/4oz GLUTEN-FREE DARK OR MILK CHOCOLATE,
    BROKEN INTO PIECES

Crème pâtissière

4 EGG YOLKS
55g/2oz/¼ CUP CASTER (SUPERFINE) SUGAR
2 TBSP GLUTEN-FREE CORNFLOUR (CORNSTARCH)
150ml/5fl oz/⅔ CUP FULL-FAT OR SEMI-SKIMMED
    (WHOLE OR LOW-FAT) MILK
150ml/5fl oz/⅔ CUP DOUBLE (HEAVY) CREAM
1 TSP VANILLA EXTRACT

Topping

650g/1lb 7oz STRAWBERRIES, HULLED, SLICED
2 TBSP STRAWBERRY JAM
GLUTEN-FREE CHOCOLATE CURLS, TO DECORATE

Cook's tip To make chocolate curls, soften some dark chocolate slightly in the microwave for 10-20 seconds then run a swivel-bladed vegetable peeler over the flat side.

A special something to share at a summery afternoon tea, barbecue or birthday celebration. These are best assembled no more than 30 minutes before serving. The chocolate-lined pastry shells can be frozen, unfilled.

1. First make the pastry: sift the flours, xanthan gum and cocoa into a mixing bowl or food processor. Mix in the sugar, then add the butter and rub in until it forms fine crumbs. Stir in the egg yolks and 1 tsp cold water, if needed, to make a soft but not sticky dough. Squeeze into a ball.

2. Cut the dough into 6 pieces. Dust your fingers lightly with rice flour, then press each piece of pastry thinly and evenly over the bottom and sides of a 10cm/4in tart tin. Press the pastry a little above the top of the tins to allow for shrinkage, and neaten the edge with scissors. Prick the bottoms with a fork and chill for 15–30 minutes.

3. Meanwhile, make the crème pâtissière: lightly whisk the egg yolks, sugar and cornflour together in a bowl until smooth. In a saucepan, bring the milk and cream just to the boil, then gradually whisk into the egg yolk mixture until smooth. Return the mixture to the saucepan and cook over a medium heat, gently whisking until very thick and smooth. Remove from the heat, stir in the vanilla, and cover the surface with a piece of crumpled and wetted baking parchment to stop a skin from forming. Leave to cool, then transfer to the fridge.

4. Preheat the oven to 190°C/375°F/Gas Mark 5. Line each pastry shell with baking parchment and dried beans. Bake for 10 minutes. Carefully remove the paper and beans and return the tarts to the oven for 4–5 minutes, until the bottoms are crisp. Leave to cool.

5. Melt the chocolate in a bowl set over a saucepan of very gently simmering water, then spoon into the pastry shells and spread all over the bottom and sides with the back of a teaspoon. Chill until set.

6. For the topping, lightly mix the strawberries and jam together and chill until needed.

7. When ready to serve, take the pastry shells out of the tins, place on serving plates and fill with the crème pâtissière. Gently stir the strawberries, then pile on to the tarts and decorate with chocolate curls.

Cook's tip Don't be tempted to use rounded tablespoons of cornflour or the crème pâtissière will be too thick. Always use level spoon measures.

GF tip Gluten-free pastry can be tricky to handle, so when making small tarts simply press the pastry thinly into the tins using your fingers. If the pastry cracks a little during baking, don't worry, as the melted chocolate will seal over the cracks.

CHRISTMAS MINCE PIES

It just wouldn't be Christmas without a warm mince pie. Traditional mincemeat usually needs to mature for a month or more, but this super-easy spiced and boozy version can be made on the day – and as it makes just enough for one batch of pies, there are no half-jars left lurking in the fridge.

MAKES 24
PREP: 40 MINUTES, PLUS 3–4 HOURS
  OR OVERNIGHT SOAKING
COOK: 15 MINUTES

Mincemeat

4 TBSP DARK RUM, BRANDY OR WHISKY
4 TBSP ORANGE JUICE
150g/5½oz MIXED DRIED FRUIT WITH CANDIED PEEL,
  ROUGHLY CHOPPED
85g/3oz READY-TO-EAT DRIED APRICOTS, DICED
85g/3oz GLACÉ (CANDIED) CHERRIES, ROUGHLY CHOPPED
85g/3oz/SCANT ½ CUP LIGHT MUSCOVADO (BROWN) SUGAR
½ TSP GROUND MIXED SPICE (PUMPKIN PIE SPICE)

Pastry

115g/4oz/¾ CUP RICE FLOUR,
  PLUS EXTRA FOR DUSTING
55g/2oz/½ CUP TAPIOCA FLOUR
55g/2oz/½ CUP GROUND ALMONDS
½ TSP XANTHAN GUM
½ TSP GROUND MIXED SPICE (PUMPKIN PIE SPICE)
FINELY GRATED ZEST OF ½ ORANGE
2 TBSP LIGHT MUSCOVADO (BROWN) SUGAR
115g/4oz/½ CUP UNSALTED BUTTER, DICED
1 EGG
MILK OR BEATEN EGG TO GLAZE
GLUTEN-FREE ICING (CONFECTIONERS') SUGAR, FOR DUSTING

1. Heat the spirit and orange juice in a saucepan until just beginning to boil, then remove from the heat and stir in the mixed dried fruit, apricots and cherries, sugar and spice. Cover and leave to soak for 3–4 hours or overnight.

2. Preheat the oven to 180°C/350°F/Gas Mark 4. To make the pastry, put the flours into a bowl or food processor, add the ground almonds, xanthan gum, spice, orange zest and sugar and mix well. Add the butter and rub in until it forms fine crumbs. Stir in the egg and mix to a soft, smooth dough.

3. Knead the dough lightly, then roll out thinly between 2 sheets of baking parchment, lightly dusted with rice flour. Using a 6cm/2½in fluted cutter, stamp out 24 circles. Press into two 12-hole mini tart tins. Fill with spoonfuls of the soaked fruit mixture.

4. Reroll the pastry trimmings and cut 24 small stars; add one to the top of each pie. Brush with a little milk or beaten egg, then bake for 15 minutes, until golden brown. Leave to stand for 15 minutes, then loosen the edges and transfer to a wire rack to cool.

5. Dust with sifted icing sugar and serve warm or cold, topped with a spoonful of brandy butter or full fat crème fraîche if you like.

GF tips
You can fill the mince pies with bought mincemeat, but check the label before buying as some brands contain wheat flour.

Although malt whisky is made with barley, it is gluten free because the distillation process removes any trace of gluten.

Cook's tip If you don't have a star cutter, cut rounds the same size as the top of the pies and make a small cut in the top for the steam to escape.

Freezing tip Make double or triple quantities and freeze in a plastic box for up to 1 month. Pack into small cellophane boxes or mini biscuit tins for a personalized Christmas gift.

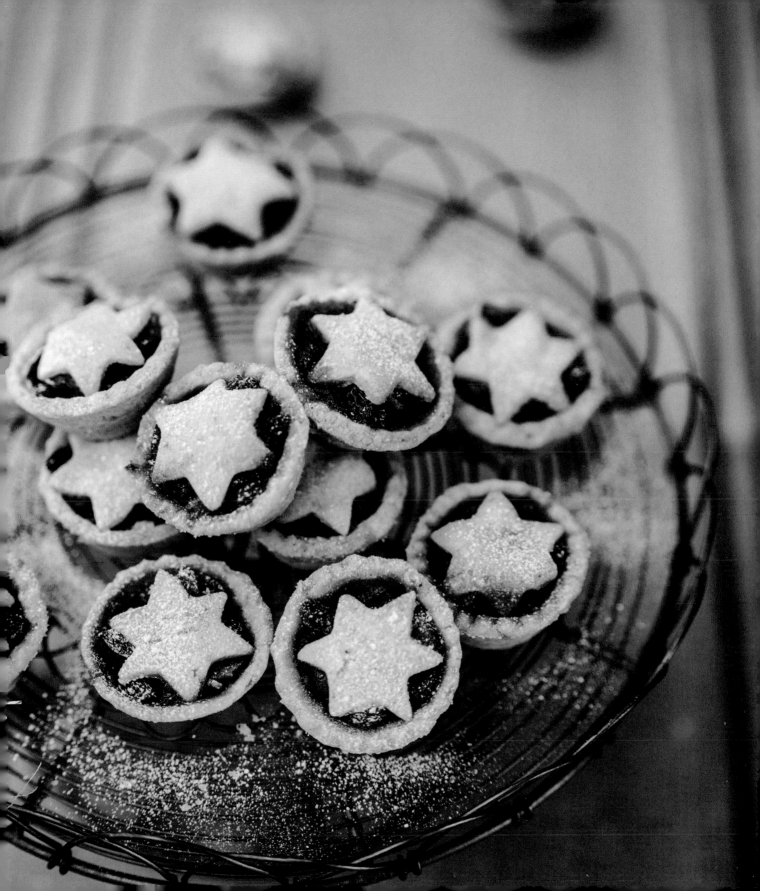

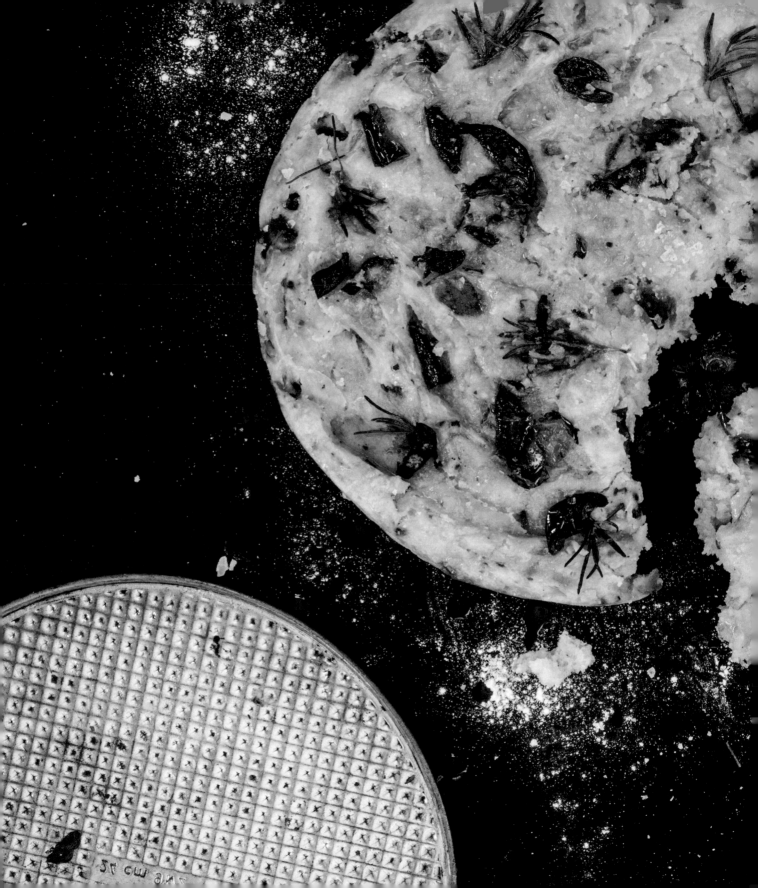

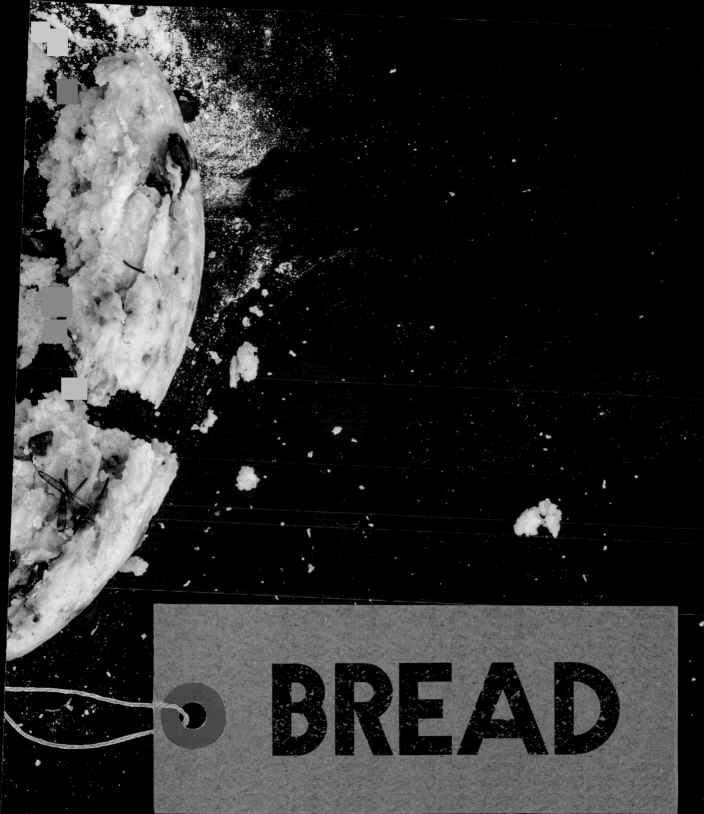

BREAD

BREAD

When you first change to a gluten-free diet, a slice of crusty bread or pizza may be one of the things that you miss the most. While nearly all supermarkets now sell gluten-free bread, it doesn't take long to make your own with some exciting combinations of flavours and textures.

Without gluten, breads are denser and more closely textured. Xanthan gum (see page 10) goes some way towards improving this by increasing the bread dough's stretch and elasticity, enabling you to make lighter bread.

In this chapter you will find breads made with a variety of flours, including some readymade flour blends, mixed with easy-blend dried yeast. They all just require one rising before being ready for baking. When you are stuck for time there are also yeast-free breads: Irish soda bread, savoury muffins or Indian flatbreads – great for breakfast or brunch, or served alongside soups and stews.

When baking bread it can be a good idea to make two loaves at a time, then enjoy one warm from the oven and freeze the second one once it has cooled. If you slice it before freezing and wrap it in a resealable bag, you will be able to take out as many slices as you need for breakfast toast or a lunchtime sandwich, as and when you need them.

Remember to keep a clearly marked gluten-free bread board to avoid cross-contamination.

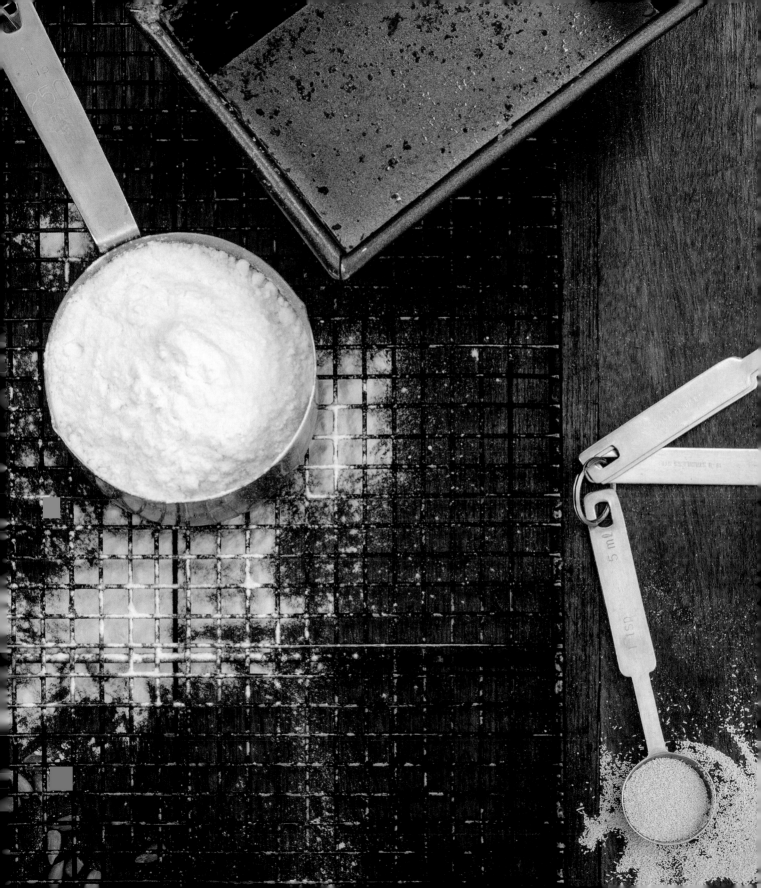

TECHNIQUES

Readymade gluten-free bread flour blends are a great standby to have in the cupboard and mean that breads made with yeast are child's play. If you plan on making your own bread more frequently, you may like to experiment with blends of different flours; remember to mix in xanthan gum to help with the stretch and lightness of your bread.

All the recipes requiring yeast are made with easy-blend dried yeast; this keeps for several months and is a handy storecupboard ingredient. There is no need to froth this type of dried yeast in water or milk; just stir it into the dry flour, salt and sugar, then mix in warm liquid to activate it. The temperature of the liquid is critical: too hot and the yeast will be killed, too cold and the yeast won't begin to work. It should feel just warm to your little finger, or 37°C/98.4°F on a cook's thermometer.

Unlike breads made with wheat flour, gluten-free flours need plenty of liquid, so that the resulting mixture is more like a thick batter than a dough. Whisk everything together, then pour the mixture into an oiled tin. Cover the top loosely with oiled clingfilm (plastic wrap) and leave in a warm place to rise for 30–60 minutes.

Gluten-free breads seem to stale more quickly than regular bread. Adding butter, olive oil or a milder-flavoured oil, such as sunflower or vegetable oil, or puréed pumpkin or butternut squash, crushed sweetcorn or chopped dried fruit all helps to keep the bread moist and fresh for longer.

To test that bread is baked, it should be golden brown and well risen. Loosen from the tin, using a knife if necessary, and knock the base lightly with your knuckles. If it sounds hollow it is ready. If not, put back in the tin or cook the bread directly on the oven shelf for 5 more minutes, then retest.

Any bread that has gone stale can be made into breadcrumbs: tear it into pieces and blitz in a food processor or blender, then store the crumbs in a resealable plastic bag in the freezer. Perfect to sprinkle over cheesy vegetable or fish gratins.

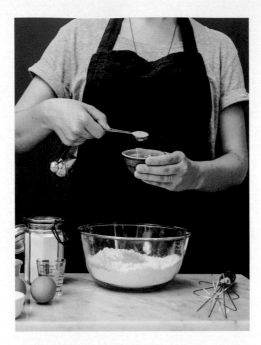

1. Put flours and xanthan gum in a large mixing bowl, add sugar, salt and easy-blend dried yeast and stir together.

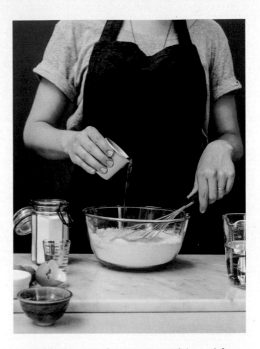

2. Add eggs and vinegar and/or oil for richness and to help keep the bread moist and fresh.

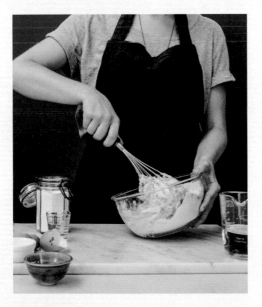

3. Whisk in warm water to make a thick batter. Gluten-free bread dough is much wetter than dough made with wheat flour.

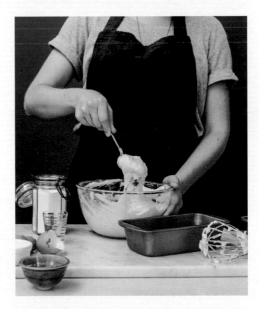

4. No kneading required, just spoon into an oiled tin, loosely cover with oiled clingfilm and leave in a warm place to rise.

SUN-DRIED TOMATO AND OLIVE FOCACCIA

SERVES 6
PREP: 30 MINUTES, PLUS 1 HOUR RISING
COOK: 30–35 MINUTES

OLIVE OIL FOR GREASING
500g/1lb 2oz/3½ CUPS GLUTEN-FREE
　WHITE BREAD FLOUR BLEND
3 TSP EASY-BLEND DRIED (ACTIVE DRY) YEAST
2 TSP CASTER (SUPERFINE) SUGAR
½ TSP SALT
ROUGHLY CRUSHED BLACK PEPPERCORNS, TO TASTE
2 SPRIGS OF FRESH ROSEMARY
2 GARLIC CLOVES, FINELY CHOPPED
55g/2oz SUN-DRIED TOMATOES
　(DRAINED WEIGHT), ROUGHLY CHOPPED
55g/2oz BLACK OLIVES, PITTED AND ROUGHLY CHOPPED
1 EGG, BEATEN
1 TSP WHITE OR RED WINE VINEGAR
6 TBSP OLIVE OIL, PLUS 4 TBSP TO FINISH
450ml/16fl oz/2 CUPS WARM WATER
COARSE SEA SALT, TO FINISH

Gluten-free dough needs to be much wetter than regular wheat-flour dough, so kneading isn't necessary, just mix, spoon into a tin and leave to rise. What could be easier?

1. Lightly oil a 25cm/10in cake tin or springform tin. Put the flour in a large mixing bowl with the yeast, sugar, salt and pepper and stir together.

2. Strip the leaves off one rosemary sprig and chop roughly – it should give about 1 tbsp – then add to the flour with the garlic, half the tomatoes and half the olives. In a small bowl, mix together the egg, vinegar and 6 tbsp oil, then add to the flour along with the warm water and whisk together to make a smooth, thick batter.

3. Spoon into the oiled tin, roughly level the top and sprinkle with the rest of the tomatoes and olives. Tear small sprigs from the remaining rosemary and press into the bread. Sprinkle with coarse salt, then cover the tin with clingfilm (plastic wrap) and put in a warm place for 50–60 minutes, until the dough is well risen. Meanwhile, preheat the oven to 220°C/425°F/Gas Mark 7.

4. Remove the clingfilm, drizzle the dough with 2 tbsp oil and bake for 30–35 minutes, until golden brown and the bread sounds hollow when tapped. Check after 20 minutes and loosely cover with foil if the rosemary is beginning to brown too much.

5. Drizzle with the remaining oil and leave to cool in the tin for 10 minutes. Turn out onto a wire rack to cool. Serve while still warm with bowls of soup, Italian antipasti or barbecued meats.

Cook's tip When making bread it is important to get the temperature of the water right: too cold and the yeast won't begin to work, too hot and the yeast will be killed. Run the water from the hot tap and when it feels just warm it is ready – or mix 150ml/5fl oz/⅔ cup boiling water with 300ml/10fl oz/1¼ cups cold water.

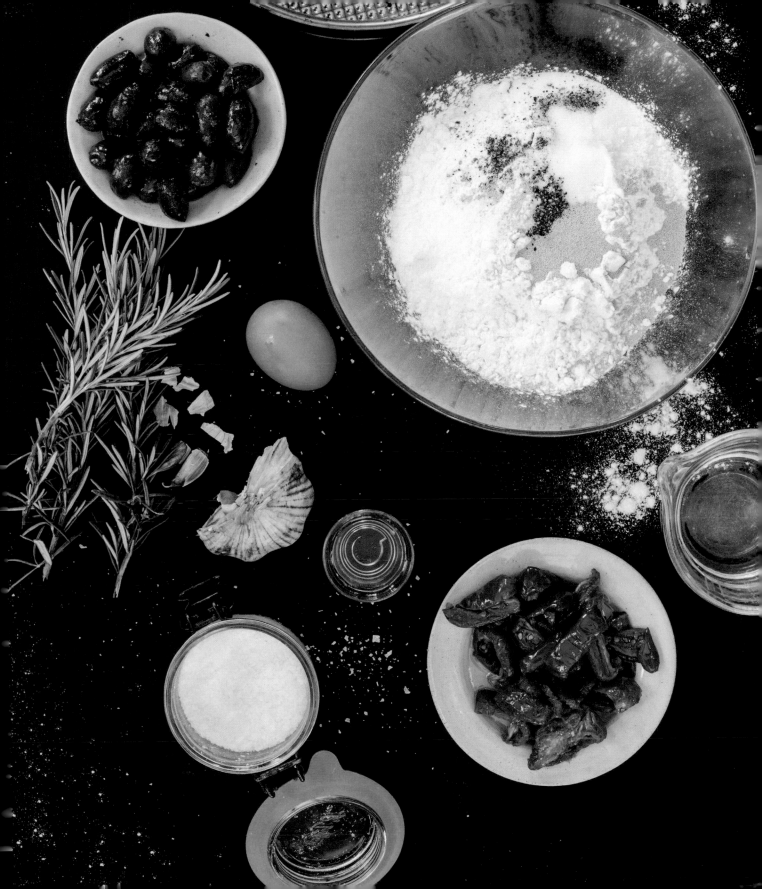

CHEESY CORN MUFFINS

MAKES 12
PREP: 15 MINUTES
COOK: 15–20 MINUTES

SUNFLOWER OIL FOR GREASING
55g/2oz/4 TBSP UNSALTED BUTTER
4 SPRING ONIONS (SCALLIONS), FINELY CHOPPED
¼ TSP DRIED CHILLI FLAKES
150g/5½oz FROZEN SWEETCORN,
    THAWED, ROUGHLY CHOPPED
150g/5½oz/1¼ CUPS FINE POLENTA (CORNMEAL)
85g/3oz/SCANT ¾ CUP TAPIOCA FLOUR
2 TSP GLUTEN-FREE BAKING POWDER
1 TSP BICARBONATE OF SODA (BAKING SODA)
1 TSP XANTHAN GUM
1 TBSP CASTER (SUPERFINE) SUGAR
115g/4oz GRUYÈRE OR CHEDDAR CHEESE, GRATED
SALT AND FRESHLY GROUND BLACK PEPPER
2 EGGS
300ml/10fl oz/1¼ CUPS BUTTERMILK

Quick and easy to put together, these American-style corn muffins, or popovers, are traditionally served with a beefy chilli, but are fab when eaten warm from the oven with grilled bacon and tomatoes for a weekend brunch or with a steaming bowl of soup for a tasty lunch.

1. Preheat the oven to 190°C/375°F/Gas Mark 5. Line a 12-hole muffin tin with paper cases or brush with a little oil, if preferred.

2. Heat a little of the butter in a small frying pan, add the spring onions and fry for 2–3 minutes, until just softened. Add the remaining butter and the chillies and heat gently until melted. Stir in the sweetcorn and remove from the heat.

3. Meanwhile, put the polenta, tapioca flour, baking powder, bicarbonate of soda, xanthan gum, sugar and cheese into a mixing bowl with plenty of salt and pepper and stir well.

4. In another bowl, beat the eggs and buttermilk together with a fork. Add to the dry ingredients, along with the sweetcorn mixture, and fork together until just mixed. Quickly spoon the mixture into the prepared muffin tin – don't worry about the spoonfuls being neat. Bake for 15–20 minutes, until golden.

5. Leave to cool in the tin for 5 minutes, then loosen the edges with a knife and remove from the tin. Serve while still hot or transfer to a wire rack to cool.

Cook's tip Instead of the buttermilk, you could use 150g/5½oz/⅔ cup low-fat plain yogurt and 150ml/5fl oz/⅔ cup semi-skimmed (low-fat) milk mixed with 1 tbsp vinegar.

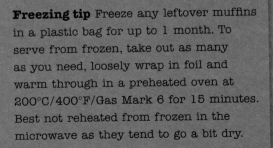

Freezing tip Freeze any leftover muffins in a plastic bag for up to 1 month. To serve from frozen, take out as many as you need, loosely wrap in foil and warm through in a preheated oven at 200°C/400°F/Gas Mark 6 for 15 minutes. Best not reheated from frozen in the microwave as they tend to go a bit dry.

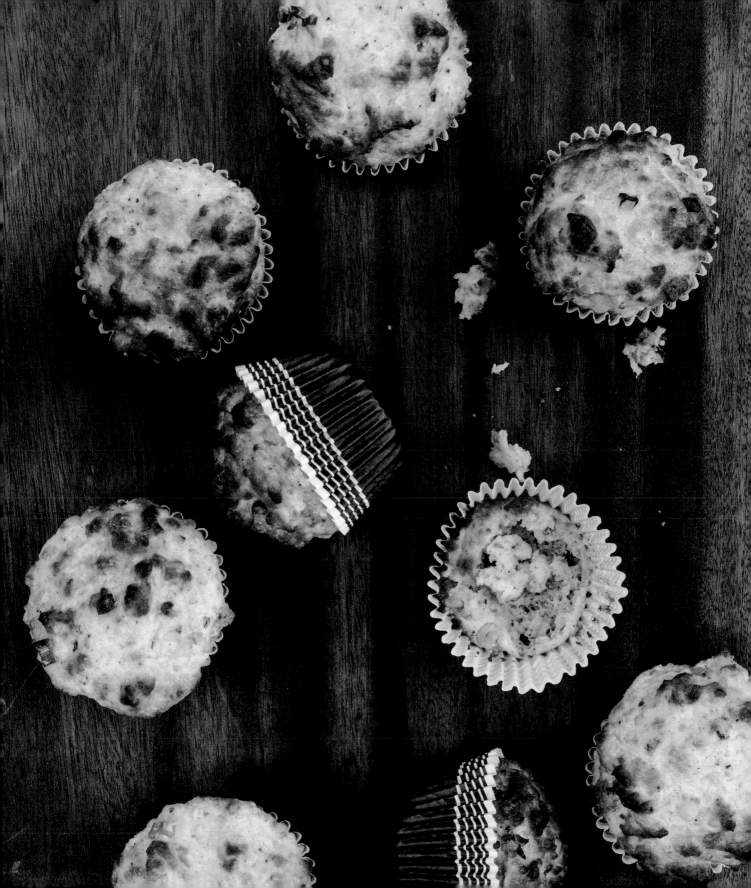

WALNUT
AND BUCKWHEAT THINS

MAKES ABOUT 40
PREP: 25 MINUTES
COOK: 10–12 MINUTES

SUNFLOWER OIL FOR GREASING
115g/4oz/1 CUP GLUTEN-FREE BUCKWHEAT FLOUR
115g/4oz/¾ CUP RICE FLOUR, PLUS EXTRA FOR DUSTING
1 TSP GLUTEN-FREE BAKING POWDER
COARSE SEA SALT AND ROUGHLY CRUSHED
    BLACK PEPPERCORNS
25g/1oz/2 TBSP LIGHT MUSCOVADO (BROWN) SUGAR
55g/2oz/4 TBSP UNSALTED BUTTER, DICED
55g/2oz/4 TBSP WHITE VEGETABLE FAT, DICED
55g/2oz/½ CUP WALNUT PIECES, ROUGHLY CHOPPED
40g/1½oz/2 TBSP HULLED SUNFLOWER SEEDS
3 TBSP SEMI-SKIMMED (LOW-FAT) MILK

Top these dainty biscuits with slices of blue cheese, or with soft goat's cheese that you have prettied up by rolling it in chopped herbs, herb flower petals or crushed peppercorns. Serve as a cheese course for a special supper, with grapes and fresh dates.

1. Preheat the oven to 200°C/400°F/Gas Mark 6. Lightly oil 2 baking sheets. Put the flours, baking powder and a pinch of salt and pepper into a mixing bowl or food processor and mix well. Stir in the sugar, then add the fats and rub in until the mixture forms fine crumbs.

2. Stir in the walnut pieces and sunflower seeds, add the milk and mix to a soft dough.

3. Lightly dust the dough and 2 sheets of baking parchment with rice flour. Lightly knead the dough, then roll out between the 2 sheets of parchment, until it is about 5mm/¼in thick.

4. Using a plain 5cm/2in round cutter, stamp out circles of dough and place on the baking sheets. Reroll the trimmings and continue stamping out until all the dough is used. Prick the dough with a fork and sprinkle with salt and pepper.

5. Bake for 10–12 minutes, until golden brown. Leave to cool on the baking sheets. Store in an airtight container for up to 4 days.

Cook's tip If you are making these in a food processor there is no need to chop the walnuts before adding – just whizz for a minute before adding the sunflower seeds and milk.

GF tip Buckwheat flour is naturally gluten-free, but always check the label as some buckwheat is grown on farms that also grow wheat and it may be cross-contaminated.

Freezing tip Pack in a plastic container, seal, label and freeze for up to 2 months. Take out as many as you need and thaw at room temperature for 1 hour.

CORIANDER AND CUMIN FLATBREADS

MAKES 12

PREP: 25 MINUTES, PLUS 30 MINUTES STANDING

COOK: 20 MINUTES

200g/7oz/GENEROUS 2 CUPS GRAM (CHICKPEA) FLOUR

150g/5½oz/1 CUP RICE FLOUR,
    PLUS EXTRA FOR DUSTING

½ TSP SALT

½ TSP XANTHAN GUM

2 GARLIC CLOVES, FINELY CHOPPED

2 TSP CUMIN SEEDS, ROUGHLY CRUSHED

HANDFUL OF FRESH CORIANDER (CILANTRO),
    FINELY CHOPPED

25g/1oz/2 TBSP UNSALTED BUTTER OR GHEE, MELTED

200–250ml/7–8fl oz/ABOUT 1 CUP WARM WATER

VEGETABLE OIL FOR FRYING

A curry night wouldn't be complete without some flatbreads. This version is made with a mix of gram (chickpea) flour and rice flour, and even though it doesn't contain any raising agent it gently puffs up when dry-fried.

1. Sift the flours, salt and xanthan gum into a bowl. Stir in the garlic, cumin and coriander, then add the butter. Gradually mix in enough warm water to make a soft, slightly sticky dough. Cover the bowl with a cloth and leave to stand for 30 minutes.

2. Cut the dough into 12 pieces. Roll out each piece between 2 sheets of baking parchment dusted with a little rice flour, to form a rough circle about 13–15cm/5–6in in diameter. Lift the soft dough off the paper and turn it from time to time to stop it sticking. Stack the rolled-out dough between smaller squares of baking parchment.

3. When you have prepared about 6 flatbreads, heat a large frying pan over a medium–high heat, pour in a little oil, then wipe out the excess with a piece of kitchen paper. Shake off any excess rice flour and cook one of the breads for a minute or two on each side until lightly puffy, with brown scorch marks. Wrap in a clean teacloth to keep warm. Wipe the pan with the oiled kitchen paper and continue baking and rolling breads until they are all cooked. Serve warm.

GF tips

Gram (chickpea) flour can sometimes be a little lumpy, so always sift before use.

If you find the breads are a little too sticky to roll out, even between the pieces of parchment, then knead in a little extra rice flour and continue.

Freezing tip Make and bake up to the end of step 4. Spread the top of each pizza with a quarter of the tomato sauce and leave to cool. Wrap the tins with clingfilm, seal and label; freeze for up to 1 month. Thaw at room temperature for 30 minutes, then add your chosen topping and bake as above.

PIZZA

MAKES 4
PREP: 30 MINUTES, PLUS 30–40 MINUTES RISING
COOK: 20–22 MINUTES

Pizza bases

500g/1lb 2oz/3½ CUPS GLUTEN-FREE
    WHITE BREAD FLOUR BLEND
3 TSP EASY-BLEND DRIED (ACTIVE DRY) YEAST
2 TSP CASTER (SUPERFINE) SUGAR
½ TSP SALT
1 EGG
1 TSP WHITE OR RED WINE VINEGAR
4 TBSP OLIVE OIL, PLUS EXTRA FOR GREASING
450ml/16fl oz/2 CUPS WARM WATER

Tomato sauce

1 TBSP OLIVE OIL, PLUS EXTRA TO FINISH
1 ONION, FINELY CHOPPED
400g CAN CHOPPED TOMATOES
1 TBSP TOMATO PURÉE (TOMATO PASTE)
HANDFUL OF FRESH BASIL, TORN INTO PIECES,
    PLUS EXTRA TO GARNISH
SALT AND FRESHLY GROUND BLACK PEPPER

Margherita topping

400g/14oz CHERRY TOMATOES, HALVED
400g/14oz MOZZARELLA CHEESE, DRAINED AND
    TORN INTO PIECES
2 TBSP OLIVE OIL, TO DRIZZLE

Younger members of the family on a gluten-free diet can miss pizza more than anything else. This simple pizza base can be frozen part-baked, then topped and finished in the oven for an easy midweek supper. Some toppings are suggested here, or add your own family favourites.

1. Lightly oil 4 x 20cm/8in round cake tins – it doesn't matter if they are not all identical.

2. To make the pizza bases, mix the flour with the yeast, sugar and salt. In a separate bowl, beat the egg, vinegar and oil together with a fork, then add to the flour and gradually whisk in the warm water to make a smooth, thick batter. Divide among the tins and spread evenly. Cover loosely with lightly oiled clingfilm (plastic wrap) and leave in a warm place for 30–40 minutes, until well risen. Preheat the oven to 220°C/425°F/Gas Mark 7.

3. Meanwhile, make the tomato sauce: heat the oil in a saucepan, add the onion and cook for 5 minutes, stirring until softened. Stir in the tomatoes, tomato purée, basil and a generous amount of salt and pepper. Simmer for 4–5 minutes, stirring from time to time, until thickened.

4. Remove the clingfilm from the pizzas. Bake for 10 minutes, until well risen and the top is firm – the bases will be quite pale at this stage.

5. Spoon the tomato sauce over the pizzas, then quickly add the halved tomato and mozzarella, sprinkle with a little salt and pepper, a drizzle of oil and a few torn basil leaves. Bake for 10–12 minutes, until the cheese is just beginning to brown. Loosen the edges of the pizza, lift out of the tins, garnish with basil, drizzle with olive oil (optional) and serve.

Cook's tip Add sliced mushrooms, red or yellow pepper, diced courgette (zucchini), and/or black olives. Or scatter with mascarpone cheese and when you take the pizzas out of the tins, add 50g/1¾oz smoked salmon per pizza, torn into pieces, and a handful of rocket (arugula) leaves.

DATE AND SUNFLOWER SEED SODA BREAD

MAKES 1 LOAF
PREP: 20 MINUTES
COOK: 35–40 MINUTES

SUNFLOWER OIL FOR GREASING
55g/2oz/GENEROUS ⅓ CUP GOLDEN FLAXSEEDS,
　　GROUND IN A BLENDER OR SPICE MILL
55g/2oz/½ CUP HEMP FLOUR
115g/4oz/¾ CUP RICE FLOUR
1 TSP BICARBONATE OF SODA (BAKING SODA)
½ TSP SALT
½ TSP XANTHAN GUM
2 TBSP LIGHT MUSCOVADO (BROWN) SUGAR
2 TBSP SUNFLOWER SEEDS, PLUS EXTRA TO DECORATE
2 TBSP PUMPKIN SEEDS, PLUS EXTRA TO DECORATE
85g/3oz PITTED DATES, CHOPPED
300ml/10fl oz/1¼ CUPS BUTTERMILK

As this Irish-style bread is not made with yeast it doesn't need to be left to rise. Serve warm, straight from the oven, with butter and jam or cold with cheese and chutney. Any leftovers taste great toasted.

1. Preheat the oven to 200°C/400°F/Gas Mark 6. Lightly grease an 18cm/7in round deep cake tin.

2. Put the ground flaxseeds in a mixing bowl, then sift in the hemp and rice flours, bicarbonate of soda, salt and xanthan gum. Stir in the sugar, sunflower seeds, pumpkin seeds and dates, then add the buttermilk and mix with a fork to make a soft dropping consistency, adding about 2 tbsp water if needed.

3. Spoon into the prepared tin, level the surface with the back of the spoon and sprinkle with a few sunflower seeds and pumpkin seeds, pressing the seeds into the top of the bread. Bake for 35–40 minutes until well risen and golden brown and the bread sounds hollow when tapped. Loosen the edge with a knife and turn out of the tin. Wrap in a clean teacloth for a soft crust or leave unwrapped for a crisp crust. Serve warm or cold.

GF tip Ground flaxseeds add a nutty taste and a moist texture. They also help to stop the bread going stale – especially in combination with the dates.
Rice flour, buckwheat flour or quinoa flour can be used instead of the hemp flour.

Cook's tips
Instead of buttermilk you could use 150g/5½oz/ ⅔cup plain yogurt and 150ml/5fl oz/⅔ cup semi-skimmed milk mixed with 1 tbsp vinegar.

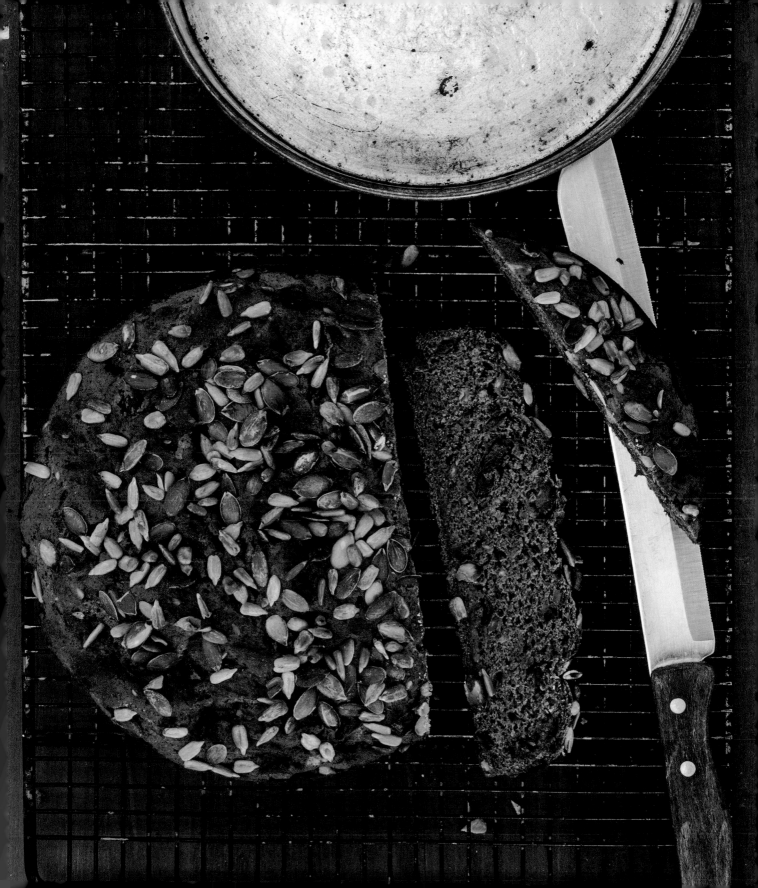

PUMPKIN AND FLAXSEED BREAD

MAKES 3 SMALL LOAVES
PREP: 15 MINUTES, PLUS 30–45 MINUTES RISING
COOK: 25–30 MINUTES

250g/9oz (PREPARED WEIGHT) PUMPKIN OR
    BUTTERNUT SQUASH, DICED
2 TSP WHITE WINE VINEGAR
2 TBSP SUNFLOWER OIL, PLUS EXTRA FOR GREASING
55g/2oz/GENEROUS ⅓ CUP GOLDEN FLAXSEEDS,
    GROUND IN A BLENDER OR SPICE MILL, PLUS 2 TBSP
    FOR SPRINKLING
650g/1lb 7oz/4⅓ CUPS GLUTEN-FREE
    WHITE BREAD FLOUR BLEND
1 TSP SALT
3 TSP CASTER (SUPERFINE) SUGAR
4 TSP EASY-BLEND DRIED (ACTIVE DRY) YEAST
2 EGGS, BEATEN
600ml/20fl oz/2½ CUPS WARM WATER
2 TBSP PUMPKIN OR SUNFLOWER SEEDS

This bread includes cooked and puréed pumpkin to keep it moist, with vitamin-boosting ground flaxseeds for added flavour. It makes three loaves: enjoy one warm from the oven and freeze two for another day.

1. Put the pumpkin in the top of a steamer, cover and cook for 10–15 minutes, or until soft. Mash or purée until smooth, then mix with the vinegar and oil. Leave to cool.

2. Lightly brush 3 x 450g/1lb loaf tins with oil.

3. Mix the flour, salt, sugar and yeast together in a large bowl, then mix in the ground flaxseeds. Add the cooled pumpkin purée and the eggs, then gradually add the water, mixing with a fork to a smooth thick batter.

4. Divide among the oiled loaf tins, put onto a baking tray, and sprinkle with the pumpkin or sunflower seeds and the extra flaxseeds. Loosely cover with oiled clingfilm (plastic wrap) and leave in a warm place to rise for 30–45 minutes, or until the bread has reached the top of the tins. Meanwhile, preheat the oven to 220°C/425°F/Gas Mark 7.

5. Remove the clingfilm and bake the bread for 25–30 minutes, until golden brown and the bread sounds hollow when tapped. Loosen the edges with a knife, then turn out onto a wire rack and leave to cool.

Freezing tip Slice one of the loaves and freeze in a plastic bag: you can take out as many slices as you need for toast in the morning – no need to thaw first.

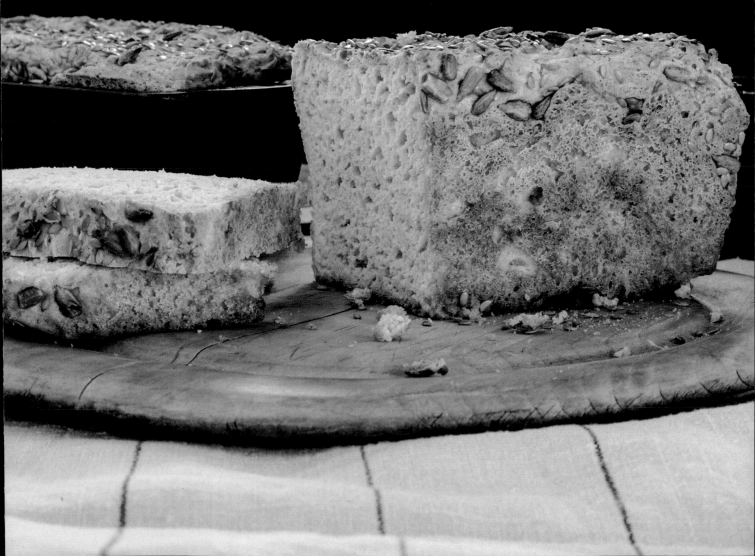

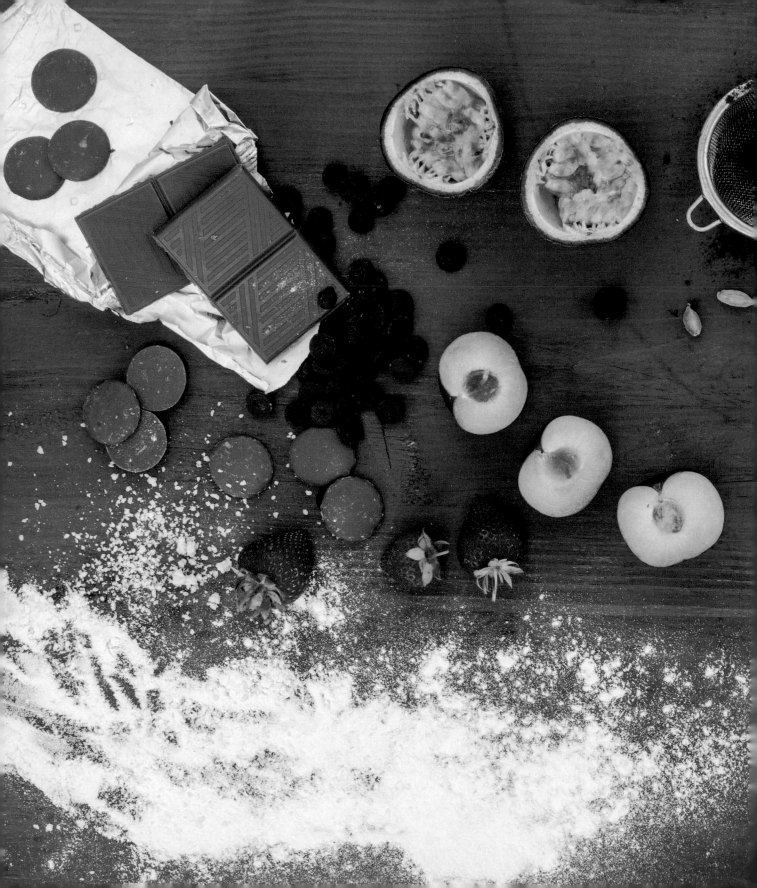

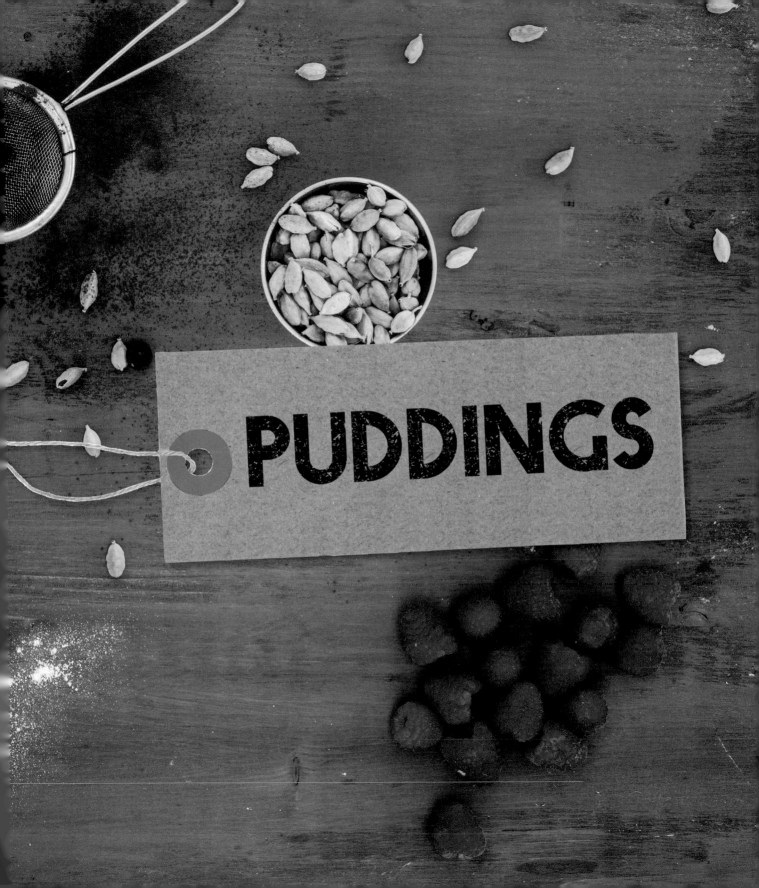

PUDDINGS

PUDDINGS

Fruit crumbles and sponge puddings are always popular – and chances are the rest of the family won't even realize what they're eating is gluten free. For a special occasion, try a gluten-free version of classic profiteroles, generously filled with cream and raspberries and drizzled with chocolate sauce. The sauce is equally good over scoops of ice cream and sliced bananas.

An easy, no-bake cheesecake is glammed up with a nutty, chocolatey, Florentine-style base and served with a boozy peach compote. Or make a more traditional base, using crushed gluten-free biscuits, or finely crushed gluten-free cornflakes, mixed with melted butter.

Meringues, in all their many guises, are naturally gluten-free. Small spooned meringues can be flavoured with a little grated gluten-free chocolate or finely chopped toasted nuts to accompany a fruity or creamy dessert. Unfilled, they keep well in an airtight tin and can be crumbled into yogurt and whipped cream speckled with summer berries for a quick Eton Mess. Larger meringue circles can be baked and layered with whipped cream and chopped fresh mint and red berries, or sweetened chestnut purée, or chocolate- or coffee-flavoured cream. As an extra indulgence, you could brush the underside of each meringue with melted chocolate and leave it to set before layering.

When summer or orchard fruits are in season, make fruit compotes with mixed or single fruits, a little water or fruit juice and some sugar or honey to sweeten, gently simmered for 5–10 minutes, until just tender. Cool, pack and freeze. Reheat and serve topped with spoonfuls of Greek yogurt or ice cream, with pancakes, or bake with a pastry or crumble topping.

At any time of year, try a creamy rice pudding, baked in the oven with a little grated nutmeg and sugar. Jazz it up by serving with poached diced dried apricots flavoured with cardamom, or with a spoonful of strawberry jam lifted with a few drops of rose water and ground cinnamon.

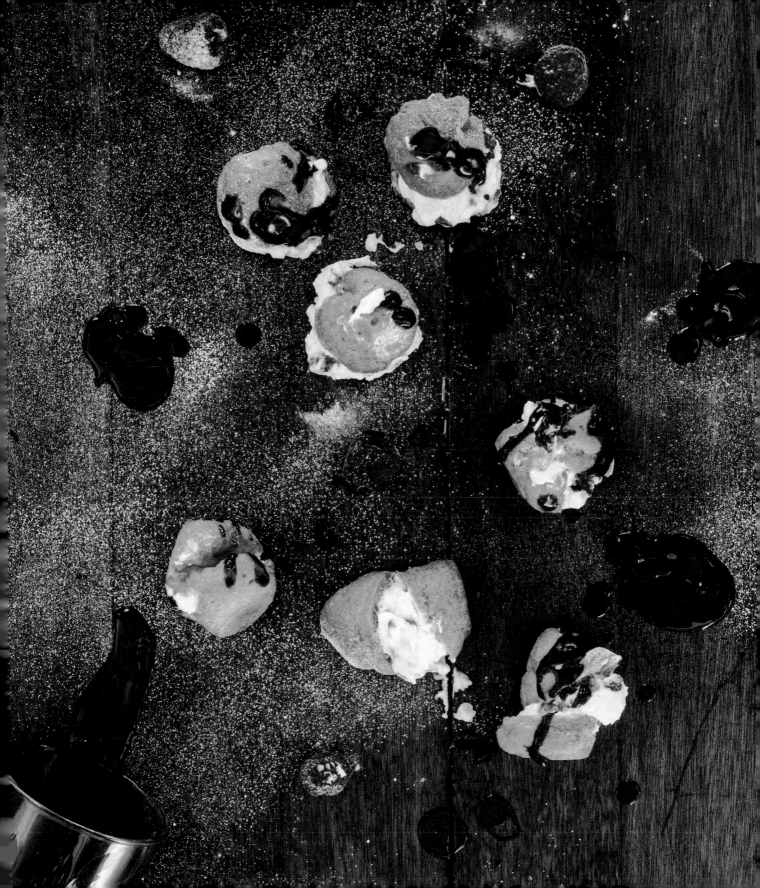

FLORENTINE CHEESECAKE
WITH MARSALA PEACHES

SERVES 6–8

PREP: 30 MINUTES, PLUS 5–6 HOURS
    OR OVERNIGHT CHILLING

COOK: 5 MINUTES

Base

SUNFLOWER OIL FOR GREASING

40g/1½oz/3 TBSP UNSALTED BUTTER

55g/2oz/½ CUP FLAKED (SLIVERED) ALMONDS,
    ROUGHLY CRUSHED

55g/2oz/SCANT ½ CUP PISTACHIO NUTS,
    ROUGHLY CHOPPED, PLUS EXTRA TO DECORATE

2 TBSP CASTER (SUPERFINE) SUGAR

85g/3oz GLUTEN-FREE DARK CHOCOLATE,
    BROKEN INTO PIECES

Cheesecake

500g/1lb 2oz/GENEROUS 2 CUPS MASCARPONE CHEESE

70g/2½oz/⅓ CUP CASTER (SUPERFINE) SUGAR

GRATED ZEST AND JUICE OF 1 UNWAXED LEMON

GRATED ZEST OF 1 ORANGE

150ml/5fl oz/⅔ CUP DOUBLE (HEAVY) CREAM

150g/5½oz/⅔ CUP GREEK-STYLE YOGURT

Marsala peaches

4 PEACHES, HALVED, STONED AND SLICED

2 TBSP CASTER (SUPERFINE) SUGAR

125ml/4fl oz/½ CUP MARSALA WINE

1 TSP GLUTEN-FREE CORNFLOUR (CORNSTARCH)

Instead of a traditional biscuit base, this Italian-inspired no-bake cheesecake has a buttery nut and chocolate base, like a Florentine, for a gluten-free alternative.

1. To make the base, lightly oil a 23cm/9in springform tin. Heat the butter in a pan, add the nuts and cook for a few minutes, until the almonds are just beginning to turn golden. Remove from the heat, add the sugar and chocolate and stir gently until melted. Tip into the oiled tin and spread evenly with the back of a spoon. Chill for 15 minutes, until just set.

2. To make the cheesecake, mix the mascarpone, sugar, all the lemon zest and half of the orange zest in a large bowl, then gradually whisk in the lemon juice until smooth. Gradually beat in the cream, until the mixture is thick, then fold in the yogurt.

3. Spoon into the tin and spread evenly, then sprinkle the remaining orange zest and a few chopped pistachios on top. Chill for 5–6 hours, or overnight.

4. For the Marsala peaches, put the peaches, sugar and Marsala in a pan, cover and cook over a low heat for about 5 minutes, or until the peaches are just beginning to soften.

5. Mix the cornflour with a little water to a smooth paste, stir into the peaches, bring to the boil and stir until thickened. Leave to cool, then store in the fridge until needed.

6. To serve, loosen the edge of the cheesecake with a knife, remove the tin sides and transfer to a serving plate. Cut into wedges and serve with the peaches.

Cook's tips

This cheesecake has a wonderfully soft texture (there's no gelatine to fiddle with), so chill it well and serve it straight from the fridge.

Instead of peaches, you could serve it with raspberries and blueberries, or a few sliced bananas dipped in lemon juice.

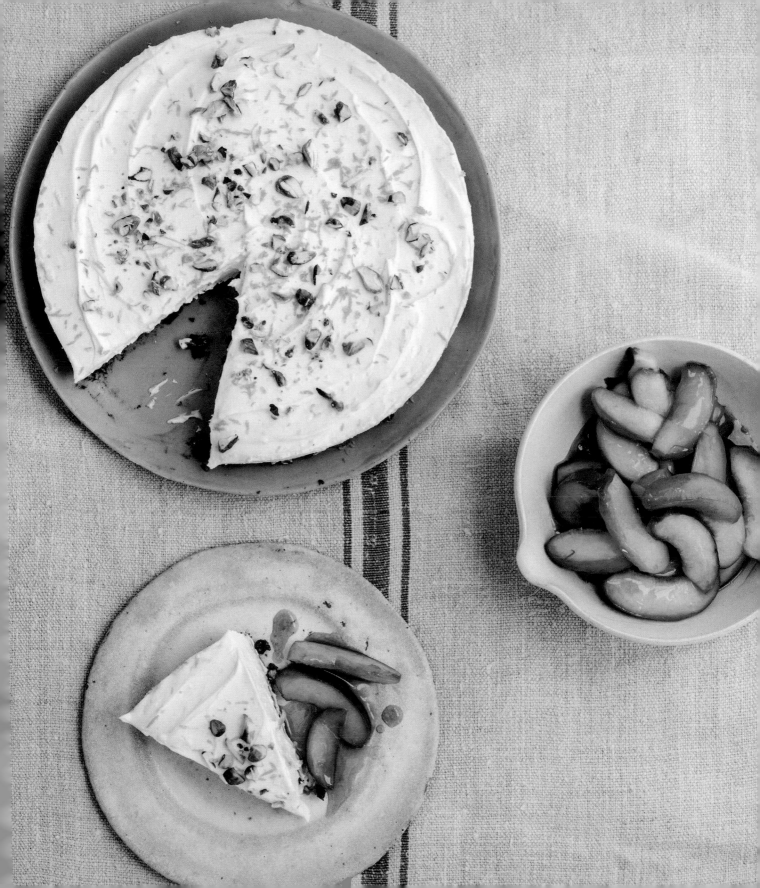

ROASTED RHUBARB AND GINGER PAVLOVA

SERVES 6
PREP: 30 MINUTES
COOK: 1¼–1½ HOURS

55g/2oz/¼ CUP LIGHT MUSCOVADO (BROWN) SUGAR
175g/6oz/GENEROUS ¾ CUP CASTER (SUPERFINE) SUGAR
1 TSP GLUTEN-FREE CORNFLOUR (CORNSTARCH)
1 TSP WHITE WINE VINEGAR
4 EGG WHITES
A FEW DROPS OF ORANGE EXTRACT

Topping

500g/1lb 2oz TRIMMED RHUBARB, THICKLY SLICED
55g/2oz/¼ CUP LIGHT MUSCOVADO (BROWN) SUGAR
2cm/¾in PIECE OF FRESH GINGER,
    PEELED AND FINELY CHOPPED
15g/½oz/1 TBSP UNSALTED BUTTER
300ml/10fl oz/1¼ CUPS DOUBLE (HEAVY) CREAM
SEEDS FROM ½ POMEGRANATE (OPTIONAL)

Pavlova figures among most people's top ten desserts. This version is made with a mixture of muscovado and caster sugar for a toffee flavour, and is topped with caramelized rhubarb.

1. Preheat the oven to 150°C/300°F/Gas Mark 2. Line a large baking sheet with baking parchment and draw a 23cm/9in circle on it, using a plate or cake tin as a guide. Mix the muscovado sugar with the caster sugar. Mix the cornflour and vinegar together in a small bowl.

2. Whisk the egg whites in a large, clean, glass bowl until stiff peaks form and the bowl can be turned upside down without the egg whites sliding. Gradually whisk in the sugars, a teaspoonful at a time, and continue whisking for a minute or two until very thick.

3. Add the cornflour mixture and orange extract and fold in gently. Spoon onto the baking sheet in soft folds within the marked circle, making a slight dip in the centre.

4. Bake for 1¼–1½ hours, or until firm to the touch and the paper can be peeled away easily from the bottom of the pavlova. Leave to cool on the paper; the pavlova will crack slightly as it cools.

5. Meanwhile, increase the oven temperature to 180°C/350°F/Gas Mark 4. Put the rhubarb in a roasting pan, sprinkle over the sugar and ginger and dot with the butter. Roast for 10 minutes, or until just tender: older, thicker stems will take a little longer than slender young stems. Leave to cool.

6. About 30 minutes before serving, remove the baking parchment and transfer the pavlova to a serving plate. Whip the cream until it forms soft swirls, fold in any juices from the rhubarb, then spoon over the pavlova and top with the rhubarb. If using, sprinkle some pomegranate seeds over the top.

Cook's tip Although best eaten on the day it is made, the pavlova base can be made a day ahead, left to cool, and kept in the fridge in a plastic container.

GF tip Always check the label: cornflour is naturally gluten free but manufacturers sometimes include wheat starch or process cornflour through machinery that is also used for wheat products.

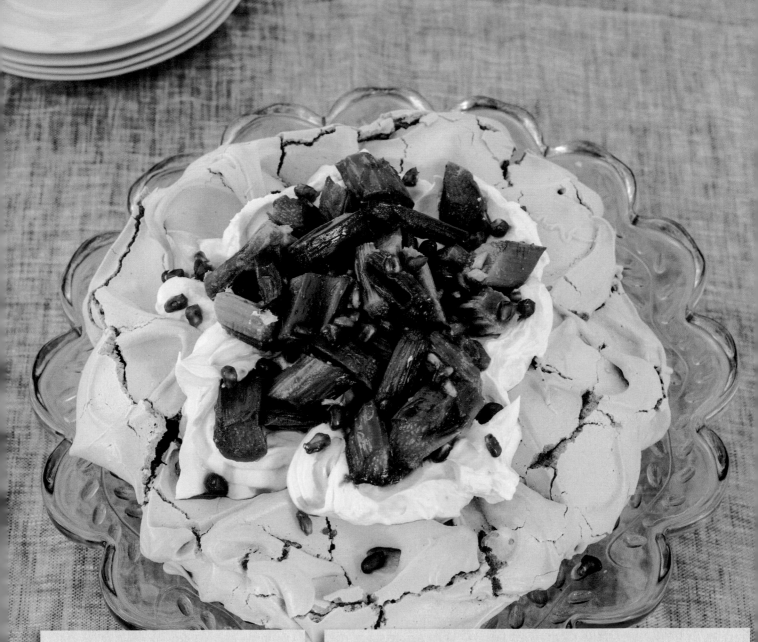

MINTED PINEAPPLE PAVLOVA

Make up the meringue as opposite but with 225g/8oz/generous 1 cup caster sugar rather than a mix of two sugars. Shape and bake as before. Top with whipped cream, then add ½ pineapple, cored, peeled and diced; sprinkle with a small bunch of finely chopped fresh mint mixed with the grated zest of 1 lime and 2 tbsp caster sugar.

INDIVIDUAL CHOCOLATE AND BANANA PAVLOVAS

Melt 100g/3½oz gluten-free dark chocolate. Make up the meringue as in steps 1 and 2. Fold in the cornflour mixture and orange extract, then add the melted chocolate and fold together very briefly, so that the meringue looks marbled. Spoon into 6 mounds on the baking sheet and spread into circles about 10cm/4in in diameter. Bake for 1–1¼ hours. Cool. Top with whipped cream and 2 bananas, thickly sliced and tossed with the juice of 1 lemon and a little diced gluten-free milk chocolate.

RASPBERRY PROFITEROLES

SERVES 4

PREP: 35 MINUTES

COOK: 15–18 MINUTES

40g/1½oz/4 TBSP RICE FLOUR
25g/1oz/3 TBSP TAPIOCA FLOUR
1 TSP GLUTEN-FREE BAKING POWDER
½ TSP BICARBONATE OF SODA (BAKING SODA)
½ TSP XANTHAN GUM
2 EGGS
½ TSP VANILLA EXTRACT
150ml/5fl oz/⅔ CUP WATER
55g/2oz/4 TBSP UNSALTED BUTTER,
   PLUS EXTRA FOR GREASING

Chocolate sauce

100g/3½oz GLUTEN-FREE DARK CHOCOLATE,
   BROKEN INTO PIECES
55g/2oz GLUTEN-FREE MILK CHOCOLATE,
   BROKEN INTO PIECES
2 TBSP GLUTEN-FREE ICING (CONFECTIONERS') SUGAR,
   PLUS EXTRA FOR DUSTING
150ml/5fl oz/⅔ CUP SEMI-SKIMMED (LOW-FAT) MILK

Filling

150ml/5fl oz/⅔ CUP DOUBLE (HEAVY) CREAM
100g/3½oz/SCANT ½ CUP GREEK-STYLE YOGURT
½ TSP VANILLA EXTRACT
150g/5½oz FRESH RASPBERRIES,
   PLUS EXTRA TO SERVE

A retro favourite that has made a bit of a comeback as we rediscover the joys of baking.

1. Preheat the oven to 200°C/400°F/Gas Mark 6. Lightly butter a large baking sheet. Sift the flours, baking powder, bicarbonate of soda and xanthan gum into a bowl. In a smaller bowl, lightly beat the eggs and vanilla together.

2. Put the water and butter in a saucepan and heat gently until the butter has melted. Bring the mixture just to the boil, then take off the heat and quickly stir in the sifted flour mixture and beat until smooth. Gradually beat in the eggs until smooth. Spoon into a piping bag fitted with a 1cm/½in plain tip.

3. Pipe 20 balls onto the baking sheet, leaving a little space between them. Bake for 12–15 minutes, until well risen, golden brown and crisp. Make a small incision in the side of each with a sharp knife to allow the steam to escape, then put them back in the oven for 2 minutes. Leave to cool on a wire rack.

4. To make the sauce, put all the ingredients in a small saucepan and heat gently, stirring until smooth. Sprinkle the surface lightly with sugar to prevent a skin from forming and set aside.

5. To fill the profiteroles, whip the cream until it forms soft swirls. Fold in the yogurt and vanilla, then crumble in the raspberries and mix briefly. Slit each profiterole and spoon in the raspberry cream. Arrange on a cake stand or in shallow serving bowls, decorate with a few raspberries and dust with sifted icing sugar. Warm the sauce and drizzle over just before serving.

CHOCOLATE ÉCLAIRS

Pipe the mixture into 5cm/2in lengths and bake for 15–18 minutes. Fill with whipped cream – flavoured with chopped preserved ginger or 1 tbsp brandy if you like. Melt 55g/2oz gluten-free dark chocolate with 15g/½oz/1 tbsp unsalted butter and 2 tbsp water in a bowl over a saucepan of gently simmering water. Take the bowl off the heat and sift in 70g/2½oz/generous ½ cup gluten-free icing sugar; stir until smooth and glossy, then spoon over the éclairs.

GF tip Gluten-free choux pastry needs additional raising agents to help it rise. The baking powder and bicarbonate of soda will begin to work as soon as they come into contact with the warm liquid, so make sure to beat in the eggs speedily and get the profiteroles into the oven as quickly as you can.

STICKY TAMARIND AND BANANA
UPSIDE-DOWN PUDDING

SERVES 8

PREP: 30 MINUTES

COOK: 45–55 MINUTES

6 TBSP GOLDEN SYRUP

1 TBSP TAMARIND PASTE

150g/5½oz/¾ CUP LIGHT MUSCOVADO (BROWN) SUGAR

3 BANANAS, PEELED

JUICE OF ½ LEMON

115g/4oz/¾ CUP RICE FLOUR

55g/2oz/½ CUP TAPIOCA FLOUR

1 TSP GLUTEN-FREE BAKING POWDER

1 TSP BICARBONATE OF SODA (BAKING SODA)

1 TSP GROUND MIXED SPICE (PUMPKIN PIE SPICE)

½ TSP GROUND GINGER

2 EGGS

3 TBSP SEMI-SKIMMED (LOW-FAT) MILK

115g/4oz/½ CUP UNSALTED BUTTER
 AT ROOM TEMPERATURE, DICED,
 PLUS EXTRA FOR GREASING

Cook's tip Tamarind paste is sold in small jars in supermarkets and Asian food shops. Check the label to ensure it is gluten-free. If you can't find it, this recipe can be made without it.

If you love sticky toffee pudding then this is sure to become a favourite. Sliced bananas baked with brown sugar balanced with the sweet and sour taste of tamarind, and topped with a spiced sponge. Serve warm from the oven with a scoop of vanilla ice cream or a drizzle of cream.

1. Preheat the oven to 160°C/325°F/Gas Mark 3. Butter a 1.5 litre/2¾ pint/7 cup rectangular baking dish or small roasting pan, about 5cm/2in deep. Line the bottom with baking parchment.

2. Spoon 3 tbsp of the golden syrup and all the tamarind over the bottom of the dish, then sprinkle over 3 tbsp of the sugar. Cut the bananas in half lengthways, coat in the lemon juice, then arrange in the dish, cut-side downwards and nestling close together.

3. Sift the flours, baking powder, bicarbonate of soda and spices into a bowl. Beat the eggs and milk together in a small bowl.

4. Cream the butter and the remaining sugar together until light and fluffy, then beat in the remaining 3 tbsp of golden syrup. Gradually beat in alternate spoonfuls of the egg and flour mixtures until all have been added and the mixture is smooth. Spoon on top of the bananas. Spread evenly, then bake for 45–55 minutes, until the sponge is well risen and the top springs back when pressed with a fingertip. Leave to stand for 10 minutes

5. Loosen the edges, cover the dish with a plate, then invert and remove the baking dish and lining paper. Cut the pudding into squares and serve immediately.

ORCHARD PUDDING

SERVES 6
PREP: 40 MINUTES
COOK: 40 MINUTES

2 PEARS, QUARTERED, CORED, PEELED AND SLICED
2 DESSERT APPLES, HALVED, CORED, PEELED AND SLICED
350g/12oz PLUMS, HALVED, STONED AND SLICED
150g/5½oz/¾ CUP CASTER (SUPERFINE) SUGAR
GRATED ZEST AND JUICE OF 1 UNWAXED LEMON
85g/3oz/GENEROUS ½ CUP RICE FLOUR
25g/1oz GLUTEN-FREE CORNFLOUR (CORNSTARCH)
1 TSP GLUTEN-FREE BAKING POWDER
115g/4oz/½ CUP UNSALTED BUTTER, AT ROOM
   TEMPERATURE, DICED, PLUS EXTRA FOR GREASING
2 EGGS
2 TBSP SEMI-SKIMMED (LOW-FAT) MILK
GLUTEN-FREE ICING (CONFECTIONERS') SUGAR, SIFTED, TO
   DECORATE

A twist on the classic British favourite 'Eve's pudding' – this version uses plums and pears as well as apples – with a lemony sponge that wraps itself around the fruit as it bakes. Serve warm, with a scoopful of vanilla ice cream, perfect after a family Sunday lunch.

1. Preheat the oven to 180°C/350°F/Gas Mark 4. Lightly butter a 1.2 litre/2 pint/5 cup round baking dish, about 4cm/1½in deep. Add the pears, apples and plums, then sprinkle with 3 tbsp of the sugar and the juice of ½ lemon. Bake, uncovered, for 15 minutes.

2. Meanwhile, mix the flours and baking powder together in a bowl and set aside. Cream the butter and the remaining caster sugar until light and fluffy.

3. Beat one egg into the creamed butter mixture, then beat in a spoonful of the flour mixture; when smooth, beat in the second egg and a little more flour, then gradually mix in the remaining flour until just smooth. Lightly mix in the milk, lemon zest and remaining lemon juice; you may find that the mixture begins to separate – quickly spoon it over the fruit and level as best you can.

4. Bake for 25 minutes, until the topping is golden and well risen. Dust with sifted icing sugar and serve warm with ice cream or pouring cream.

Cook's tip Instead of apples, pears and plums, try peaches, plums and raspberries, apples, pears and blackberries, or use just one fruit.

PLUM STRAWBERRY AND COCONUT CRUMBLE

SERVES 4

PREP: 20 MINUTES

COOK: 40 MINUTES

550g/1lb 4oz PLUMS, QUARTERED AND STONED

400g/14oz STRAWBERRIES, HULLED, HALVED OR THICKLY SLICED IF LARGE

25g/1oz/2 TBSP CASTER (SUPERFINE) SUGAR

2 TBSP WATER

Crumble topping

85g/3oz/GENEROUS ½ CUP BROWN RICE FLOUR

55g/2oz/½ CUP MILLET FLAKES

70g/2½oz/5 TBSP UNSALTED BUTTER, DICED

55g/2oz/4 TBSP CASTER (SUPERFINE) SUGAR

55g/2oz/GENEROUS ½ CUP DESICCATED COCONUT

Coconut custard

4 EGG YOLKS

40g/1½oz/3 TBSP CASTER (SUPERFINE) SUGAR

400ml CAN COCONUT MILK

FINELY GRATED ZEST OF 1 LIME

Crumble topping is quick and easy to make and freezes well, so why not multiply the recipe, pack into plastic containers and freeze? Use the crumble straight from the freezer – without thawing – to top partly cooked plums and strawberries, apples and blackberries, or your own favourite fruit combination, then bake.

1. Preheat the oven to 180°C/350°F/Gas Mark 4. Put the fruit in a 1.7 litre/3 pint/8 cup shallow baking dish. Sprinkle over the sugar and water and bake, uncovered, for 10 minutes to soften the fruit.

2. To make the crumble topping, put the rice flour and millet flakes in a bowl, add the butter and rub in until it forms fine crumbs. Stir in the sugar and coconut and sprinkle over the fruit.

3. Bake for 30 minutes – check after 20 minutes and cover loosely with foil if the coconut seems to be browning too quickly.

4. While the crumble cooks, make the custard by whisking the egg yolks and sugar together briefly, until smooth. Pour the coconut milk into a saucepan, bring just to the boil, then gradually whisk into the yolk mixture. Add the lime zest, return the mixture to the saucepan and cook over a low heat, stirring with a wooden spoon, until the custard just coats the back of the spoon. Serve hot, with the crumble.

Cook's tip Don't be tempted to try and speed up the custard cooking time by raising the temperature. If it is too hot the eggs will curdle and spoil the custard.

GF tip You could use oats instead of millet flakes, but not all coeliacs can tolerate them, so if you are very sensitive to gluten it is best to avoid them. Read labels carefully as oats can become cross-contaminated during production and are not guaranteed to be gluten free.

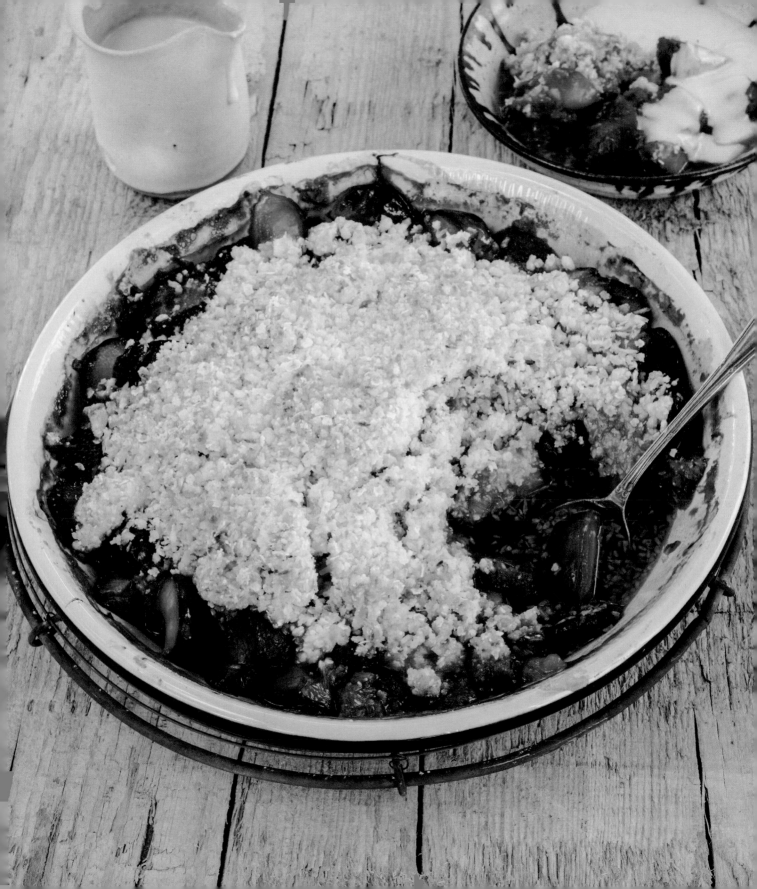

CHOCOLATE AND CARDAMOM SPONGE PUDDINGS
WITH CHILLI CHOCOLATE SAUCE

SERVES 6

PREP: 15 MINUTES

COOK: 20 MINUTES

115g/4oz READY-TO-EAT PRUNES, CHOPPED

125ml/4fl oz/½ CUP WATER

3 GREEN CARDAMOM PODS, CRUSHED

½ TSP GROUND CINNAMON

125ml/4fl oz/½ CUP SUNFLOWER OIL,
    PLUS EXTRA FOR GREASING

2 EGGS

115g/4oz/GENEROUS ½ CUP LIGHT MUSCOVADO
    (BROWN) SUGAR

115g/4oz/SCANT 1 CUP SELF-RAISING GLUTEN-FREE
    FLOUR BLEND

15g/½oz UNSWEETENED COCOA POWDER, PLUS EXTRA
    FOR DUSTING

SIFTED GLUTEN-FREE ICING (CONFECTIONERS') SUGAR
    FOR DUSTING

MASCARPONE CHEESE FLAVOURED WITH A LITTLE VANILLA
    EXTRACT, TO SERVE

Chilli chocolate sauce

115g/4oz GLUTEN-FREE DARK CHOCOLATE,
    BROKEN INTO PIECES

2 TBSP LIGHT MUSCOVADO (BROWN) SUGAR

¼ TSP GROUND CINNAMON

PINCH OF CHILLI POWDER

150ml/5fl oz/⅔ CUP SEMI-SKIMMED (LOW-FAT) MILK

Dark, rich and wonderfully comforting. Hot chocolatey sponge drizzled with a spiced sauce that contrasts with the cold creaminess of vanilla-flavoured mascarpone or ice cream.

1. Preheat the oven to 180°C/350°F/Gas Mark 4. Lightly oil 6 x 200ml/7fl oz/¾ cup individual metal pudding moulds. Put the prunes, water, cardamom pods and their black seeds and ground cinnamon in a small saucepan, bring the water to the boil, then simmer for 5 minutes.

2. Discard the cardamom pods, then purée the mixture in a blender and spoon into a bowl. Whisk in the oil, eggs and muscovado sugar, then stir in the flour and cocoa until smooth.

3. Divide among the pudding moulds, place on a baking sheet and bake, uncovered, for 15 minutes, until well risen.

4. Meanwhile, make the sauce: put the chocolate, sugar, cinnamon and chilli in a small saucepan. Pour in the milk and heat gently, stirring, until the chocolate has melted and the sauce is smooth and glossy.

5. Loosen the edges of the puddings, turn out of the tins into shallow serving bowls and dust lightly with cocoa and icing sugar. Add a spoonful of vanilla-flavoured mascarpone to each bowl, drizzle with the warm sauce and serve immediately.

Cook's tip Prunes help to keep the sponge puddings moist. Mashed sweet potato could be used instead.

GF tip A commercial flour blend, with the raising agent already added, is a handy standby. If you have time, experiment with making your own gluten-free flour blends, using combinations of tapioca flour, cornflour, rice flour, sorghum flour and potato starch.

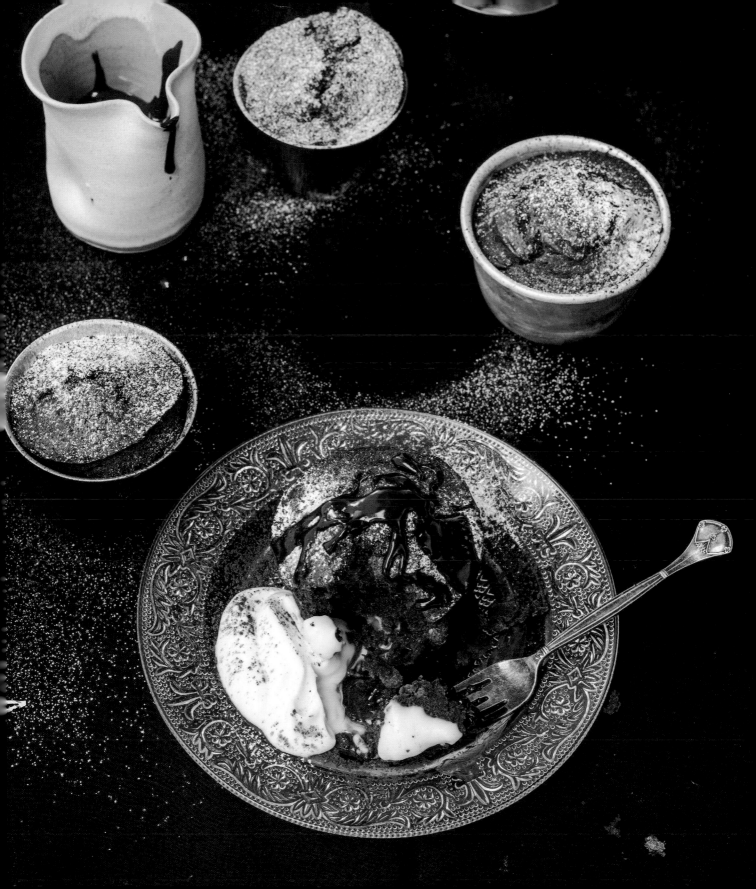

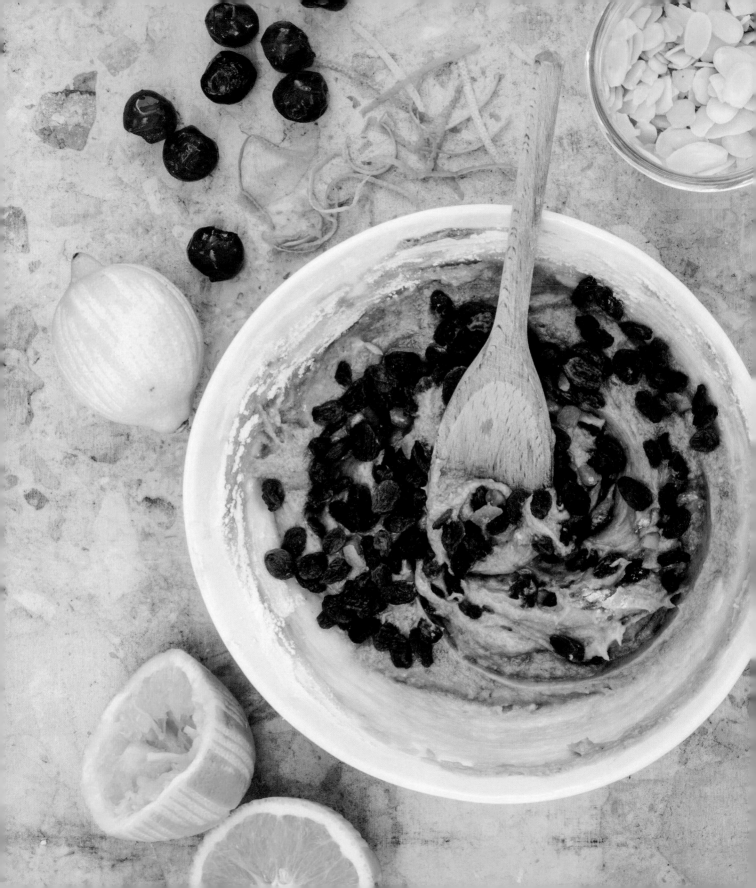

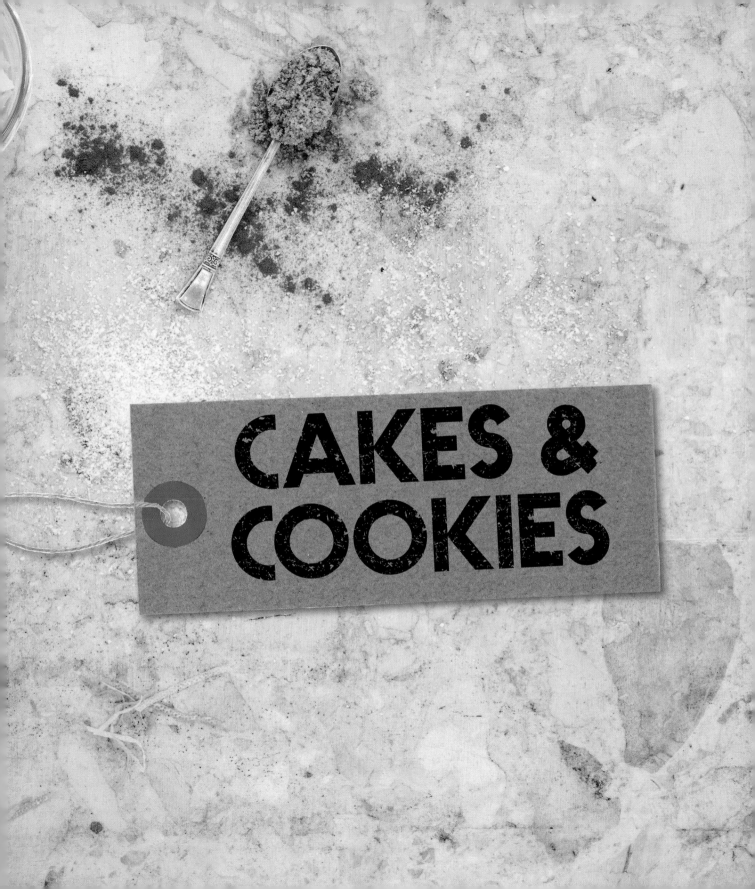

CAKES &
COOKIES

CAKES & COOKIES

When it comes to satisfying your sweet tooth, do you choose a crisp shortbread, a light lemon drizzle cake or a gooey chocolate brownie? A delicious range of cakes and cookies can be made easily without gluten, and those tucking into them will have no idea that they are created with a special diet in mind.

For great tasting cakes, a combination of tapioca flour (milled from the cassava root) and finely ground rice flour generally produces the lightest and best results – or use a ready-prepared gluten-free flour blend that includes the raising agent, for ease. Read the label before buying baking powder, as not all brands are gluten-free. Different types of flour absorb different amounts of liquid, so try to avoid swapping one flour for another in recipes.

Butter, sugar, eggs and nuts are all naturally gluten-free. Ground almonds, hazelnuts or pistachio nuts keep cakes moist and improve storage life, but can be expensive. For a budget alternative add golden linseeds or sunflower seeds – grind them in the blender shortly before using them.

When buying chocolate or cocoa, read the labels carefully as not all brands are gluten free – some may be produced on machines that also process foods that contain gluten.

When making individual cakes or muffins it can be handy to freeze some for another day. Take out as many as you need and add to a lunchbox while still frozen; by lunchtime they will be ready to eat.

Sandwich cakes can be frozen, unfilled. Wrap well with foil or clingfilm (plastic wrap) and pack into a plastic container to protect them from damage. Thaw at room temperature and fill when needed.

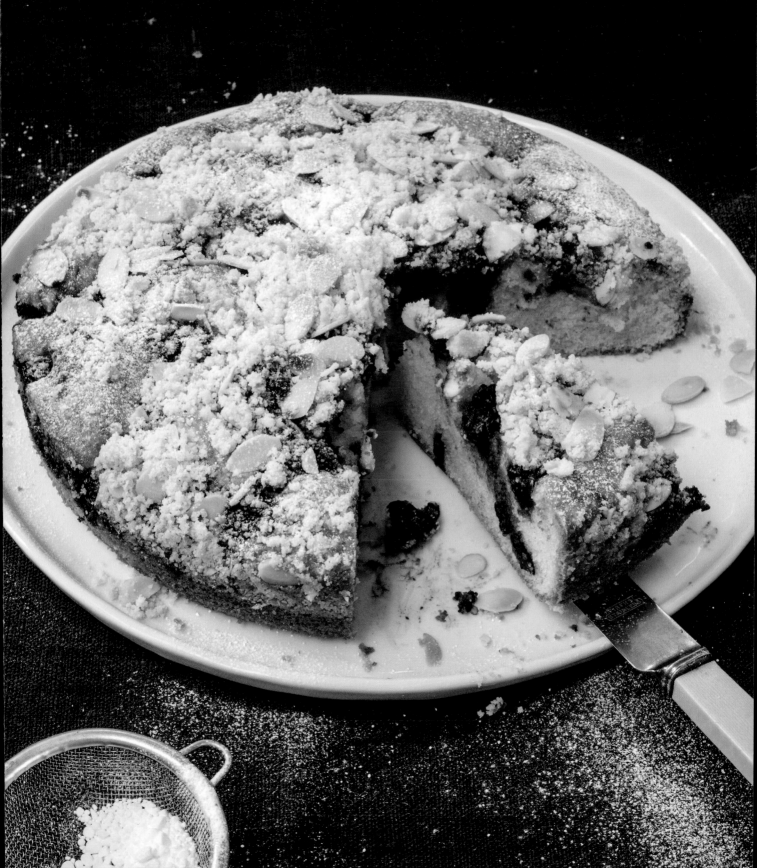

TECHNIQUES

Many cakes are made by the creaming method shown opposite, in which butter and sugar are beaten with a wooden spoon or with an electric mixer until pale and fluffy, then eggs and flours are gradually mixed in. Other cakes rely on the air that is whisked into the eggs to help them rise; these need a very gentle approach when folding in flour so that as much air as possible is held within the delicate mixture.

When you need a cake in a hurry, American-style muffins are super easy: simply mix all the dry ingredients in one bowl and the wet ones in a jug, then add the wet to the dry and fork together. The less you beat the mixture the lighter the muffins will be – it doesn't matter if there are a few specks of flour not fully mixed in. Shortbread can be blitzed together in seconds in a food processor, or rubbed in by hand; flavour with grated orange or lemon zest, chopped rosemary or lavender petals, or a few chocolate chips.

When baking, ingredients must be measured accurately on kitchen scales. Measuring spoons are essential for ingredients used in small quantities, such as spices, baking powder and xanthan gum; always use level rather than rounded spoonfuls. If possible, use the size of cake tin mentioned in the recipe. If the tin is larger the cake will be thinner and will cook more quickly; if smaller, the cake will probably bubble over the top. Brush the tins evenly with a little oil and line the base with non-stick baking paper (baking parchment) so that the cake will come out of the tin easily.

Always preheat the oven so that it is the correct temperature when the cake goes in. Keep a watchful eye on the cake during cooking as ovens do vary. Check halfway through cooking and cover the top loosely with foil if it seems to be browning too quickly.

To check if your cake is cooked, insert a fine skewer into the centre of a deep cake such as a fruit cake or ginger cake. If the skewer comes out cleanly the cake is ready; if not, cook for 5–10 minutes more and then retest. For thinner sandwich-style cakes, lightly press the centre of one of the cakes with a fingertip. The cake will spring back when ready.

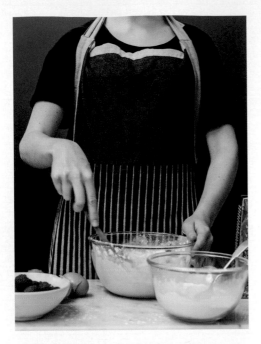

1. Cream butter and sugar together until light and fluffy. The more you beat, the more air you will incorporate.

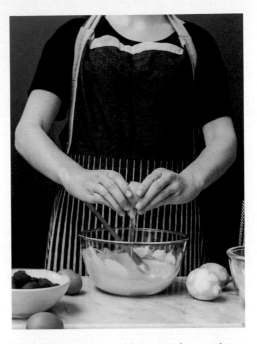

2. Add one egg and beat until smooth. Don't be tempted to add the eggs all at once or the cake mixture will curdle.

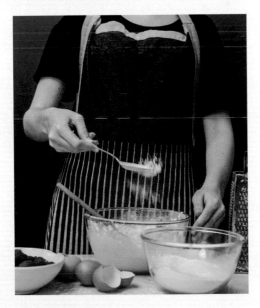

3. Gradually beat in alternate spoonfuls of the flour blend and the remaining eggs, beating well after each addition.

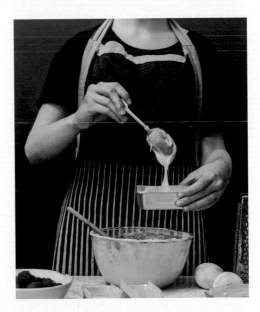

4. Spoon the cake mixture into oiled and lined tins. Level the surface of each cake with a round-bladed knife.

CELEBRATION CHOCOLATE CAKE

MAKES 10 SLICES

PREP: 30 MINUTES

COOK: 40 MINUTES

25g/1oz/3 TBSP UNSWEETENED COCOA POWDER

1 TSP XANTHAN GUM

1 TSP GLUTEN-FREE BAKING POWDER

55g/2oz/½ CUP TAPIOCA FLOUR

4 EGGS

115g/4oz/GENEROUS ½ CUP CASTER (SUPERFINE) SUGAR

55g/2oz/½ CUP GROUND ALMONDS

To decorate

400ml/14fl oz/1¾ CUPS DOUBLE (HEAVY) CREAM

1 TSP VANILLA EXTRACT

2 TBSP GLUTEN-FREE ICING (CONFECTIONERS') SUGAR

225g/8oz/SCANT 2 CUPS RASPBERRIES

350g/12oz STRAWBERRIES, HALVED IF SMALL,
    SLICED IF LARGE

UNSWEETENED COCOA POWDER, SIFTED, OR GLUTEN-FREE
    DARK CHOCOLATE, GRATED

Cook's tip If you have a hand-held electric whisk, set the bowl of eggs and sugar over a saucepan of gently simmering water and whisk until thick. When the mixture is thick enough to leave a trail, take the bowl off the heat and fold in the cocoa mixture and almonds.

Dress up this light-as-air chocolate cake with either sifted unsweetened cocoa, drizzled melted chocolate, chocolate shavings made with a vegetable peeler, sugar sprinkles, sparklers or candles – get creative!

1. Preheat the oven to 180°C/350°F/Gas Mark 4. Grease a 23cm/9in springform tin with sunflower oil and line the bottom with baking parchment. Sift the cocoa, xanthan gum and baking powder into a bowl, then stir in the tapioca flour.

2. Crack the eggs into the bowl of an electric mixer, add the sugar and beat for 5–10 minutes, until very thick and pale – when the whisk is lifted the mixture should leave a trail that remains on the surface for a few seconds.

3. Very gently fold in the cocoa mixture. Add the ground almonds and gently cut in and fold with a large metal spoon. Take great care not to knock out the air.

4. Pour the mixture into the prepared tin, lightly smooth the top, then bake for 20–25 minutes, until well risen and a skewer inserted into the centre of the cake comes out clean. Leave to cool in the tin for 15 minutes, then loosen the edge, remove the sides and bottom of the tin and transfer the cake to a wire rack to cool completely.

5. When cold, peel away the lining paper and cut the cake in half horizontally. Put one half on a large serving plate.

6. Whip the cream until it forms soft peaks, then fold in the vanilla and icing sugar. Spoon half over the cake and scatter over half the berries. Cover with the other half of the cake, then spoon over the remaining cream and decorate with the remaining fruit. Sprinkle over a little cocoa, add candles and serve.

Freezing tip Cut the cooked (unfilled) cake in half and sandwich together with a square of baking parchment or foil in between, wrap in foil and freeze for up to 1 month. Thaw for an hour or so at room temperature, then separate the two halves and fill with the cream and fruit.

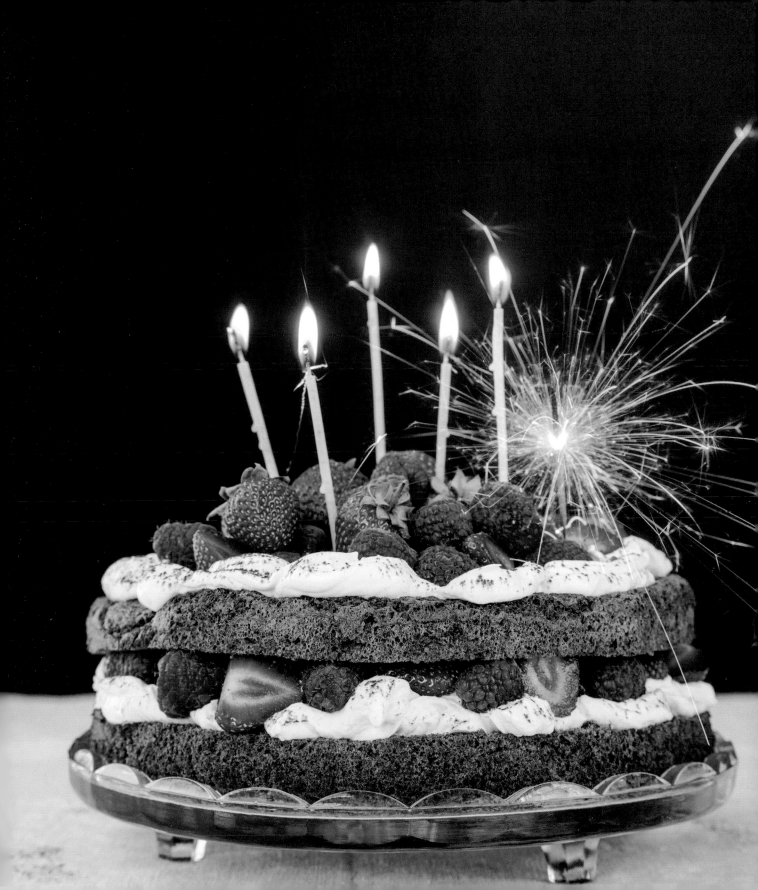

BANANA CRANBERRY AND POLENTA CAKE

MAKES 10 SLICES

PREP: 40 MINUTES, PLUS 10 MINUTES COOLING

COOK: 1 HOUR

150g/5½oz/1¼ CUPS FINE POLENTA (CORNMEAL)

85g/3oz/SCANT ¾ CUP TAPIOCA FLOUR

1 TSP GLUTEN-FREE BAKING POWDER

½ TSP BICARBONATE OF SODA (BAKING SODA)

1 TSP XANTHAN GUM

115g/4oz/½ CUP UNSALTED BUTTER,
    AT ROOM TEMPERATURE, DICED,
    PLUS EXTRA FOR GREASING

115g/4oz/GENEROUS ½ CUP SOFT LIGHT BROWN SUGAR

2 EGGS

2 RIPE BANANAS, 400g/14oz WEIGHED WITH SKINS ON,
    PEELED

GRATED ZEST AND JUICE OF 1 SMALL ORANGE

75g/2¾oz/GENEROUS ½ CUP DRIED CRANBERRIES

115g/4oz/1 CUP GLUTEN-FREE ICING (CONFECTIONERS')
    SUGAR

Cook's tip If you have a food processor, there's no need to mash the bananas, just break into pieces, add with the orange zest and blitz. Add the cranberries at the end and blitz very briefly so that they stay in large pieces.

Make the most of those brown-speckled bananas in the fruit bowl as a base for this cake. It keeps for up to three days in an airtight container, or can be frozen without the icing.

1. Preheat the oven to 160°C/325°F/Gas Mark 3. Grease a 900g/2lb loaf tin and line the long sides and bottom with a piece of baking parchment.

2. Put the polenta, tapioca flour, baking powder, bicarbonate of soda and xanthan gum into a bowl and mix well. Cream the butter and brown sugar together in a large bowl until light and fluffy. Beat one egg into the mixture, add a little of the flour mixture and beat until smooth, then add the second egg and the remaining flour and mix well.

3. Mash the bananas with a fork, then stir into the cake mixture, together with the orange zest. Reserve a few cranberries to decorate, and stir the rest into the cake mixture.

4. Spoon into the prepared tin, roughly level the top, then bake for about 1 hour, until well risen, the top has cracked and a skewer inserted into the centre of the cake comes out clean. Check after 40 minutes and if the cake seems to be browning too quickly, cover the top loosely with foil.

5. Leave to cool in the tin for 10 minutes, then loosen the edges and turn out onto a wire rack to cool completely.

6. To decorate, sift the icing sugar into a bowl and stir in 3–4 teaspoons of orange juice to make a smooth icing. Peel back the lining paper sides and drizzle the icing over the cake. Roughly chop the remaining cranberries and scatter over the top. Leave for 30 minutes for the icing to set, then discard the lining paper, transfer the cake to a plate and serve.

RICH FRUIT CAKE

MAKES 20 SLICES

PREP: 40 MINUTES, PLUS 2–3 HOURS
    OR OVERNIGHT SOAKING

COOK: 2½–3 HOURS

150ml/5fl oz/⅔ CUP BRANDY, WHISKY OR RUM,
    PLUS 2–3 TBSP TO FINISH

GRATED ZEST AND JUICE OF ½ UNWAXED LEMON

GRATED ZEST AND JUICE OF ½ ORANGE

650g/1lb 7oz MIXED DRIED FRUIT
    WITH MIXED (CANDIED) PEEL

115g/4oz READY-TO-EAT DRIED APRICOTS,
    ROUGHLY CHOPPED

115g/4oz PITTED DATES OR DRIED FIGS,
    ROUGHLY CHOPPED

115g/4oz GLACÉ (CANDIED) CHERRIES, QUARTERED

115g/4oz/¾ CUP RICE FLOUR

115g/4oz/SCANT 1 CUP TAPIOCA FLOUR

1 TSP GROUND MIXED SPICE (PUMPKIN PIE SPICE)

1 TSP GROUND CINNAMON

1 TSP XANTHAN GUM

225g/8oz/1 CUP UNSALTED BUTTER,
    AT ROOM TEMPERATURE, DICED

225g/8oz/GENEROUS 1 CUP DARK MUSCOVADO
    (BROWN) SUGAR

4 EGGS

55g/2oz/SCANT ½ CUP BLANCHED ALMONDS, HALVED

1 TBSP CHOPPED GLACÉ (CANDIED) GINGER

Topping

40g/1½oz/5 TBSP BLANCHED ALMONDS

40g/1½oz/6 TBSP PECAN HALVES

55g/2oz GLACÉ (CANDIED) CHERRIES, HALVED

There's no reason why a special celebration cake should be out of bounds: no one need know that this is made with gluten-free flour. The mixture can be scaled up to make a larger cake, even a wedding cake. This will keep for up to one month in a cake tin.

1. Pour the spirit into a saucepan, add the lemon and orange zests and juices and bring just to the boil. Remove from the heat and stir in the mixed dried fruit, apricots, dates or figs and glacé cherries and mix well. Cover and leave to soak for 2–3 hours or overnight.

2. Preheat the oven to 150°C/300°F/Gas Mark 2. Line the bottom and sides of a 20cm/8in round deep cake tin with a double thickness of baking parchment. Mix the flours, spices and xanthan gum together in a bowl.

3. Cream the butter and sugar together in a large bowl using an electric mixer. Add one egg and beat well, then add a spoonful of the spiced flour and beat again; continue adding eggs and flour alternately, then add the remaining flour beating until the mixture is smooth.

4. Add the almonds and ginger, then gradually mix in the soaked fruit and any liquid. Mix well, then spoon the mixture into the prepared tin and press down to level the surface. Decorate the top with rows of almonds, pecans and cherries.

5. Bake for 2½–3 hours, or until a skewer inserted into the centre of the cake comes out clean. Check after 1½ hours and cover the top of the cake loosely with foil if it seems to be browning too quickly. Leave to cool in the tin for 1 hour.

6. Remove from the tin and leave to cool completely. When cold, remove the paper, pierce the cake with a skewer and drizzle with 2–3 tbsp of spirit. Slice and serve.

Cook's tip For an iced cake, omit the nut and cherry decoration in step 4. When cooked and cooled, spread thinly with 4 tbsp warmed, sieved apricot jam mixed with 1 tbsp water. Cover with 700g/1lb 9oz gluten-free marzipan and then 700g/1lb 9oz ready-to-roll gluten-free icing.

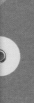

Freezing tip Cut the cooled cake into wedges and wrap each piece in clingfilm; freeze for up to 2 months. Thaw at room temperature for 2 hours. You may find it easier to make it in an 18cm/7in square tin so that it is easier to slice.

APPLE SAUCE CAKE

MAKES 8 SLICES
PREP: 30 MINUTES
COOK: 35 MINUTES

550g/1lb 4oz GRANNY SMITH APPLES,
    QUARTERED, CORED, PEELED AND DICED
125ml/4fl oz/½ CUP DRY CIDER
175g/6oz/GENEROUS ¾ CUP LIGHT MUSCOVADO
    (BROWN) SUGAR
115g/4oz/¾ CUP RICE FLOUR
115g/4oz/SCANT 1 CUP TAPIOCA FLOUR
2 TSP GLUTEN-FREE BAKING POWDER
1 TSP XANTHAN GUM
85g/3oz/6 TBSP UNSALTED BUTTER, MELTED,
    PLUS EXTRA FOR BUTTERING
2 EGGS
200ml/7fl oz/¾ CUP DOUBLE (HEAVY) CREAM
GLUTEN-FREE ICING (CONFECTIONERS') SUGAR, SIFTED,
    TO DECORATE

The apple purée in this cake mixture adds a wonderful moistness and flavour. Sandwich the cakes with more purée and soft folds of whipped cream and enjoy with a leisurely cup of tea.

1. Put the apples, cider and 55g/2oz/¼ cup of the sugar in a saucepan, bring just to the boil, then simmer for 15 minutes, stirring from time to time, until the apples are soft and the cider has mostly evaporated. Mash the apples and leave to cool.

2. Preheat the oven to 180°C/350°F/Gas Mark 4. Butter and line the bottoms of 2 x 20cm/8in round shallow cake tins.

3. Put the flours, baking powder and xanthan gum in a bowl with the remaining sugar and mix well. Add the melted butter, eggs and 300g/10½oz of the apple purée and whisk together until smooth.

4. Divide the mixture between the tins, smooth the tops and bake for about 20 minutes, until golden brown and the tops spring back when pressed with a fingertip. Leave to cool in the tins for 5 minutes, then loosen the edges with a knife, turn out onto a wire rack and peel off the paper. Leave to cool completely.

5. To serve, transfer one cake to a serving plate. Lightly whip the cream until it just holds its shape, then spread over the cake. Top with spoonfuls of the remaining apple purée, then cover with the remaining cake. Dust the top lightly with icing sugar and serve.

Cook's tip Cider is great in cooking – it doesn't matter if it has gone a bit flat. Store it in the fridge in a screwtop bottle. If you'd rather not use cider, then add the same amount of water or apple juice.

Freezing tip Wrap the cakes in foil and spoon the remaining apple purée into a small plastic box. Seal, label and freeze for up to 2 months. Thaw at room temperature for 3–4 hours. Stir the apple purée before using it to sandwich the cakes together with freshly whipped cream.

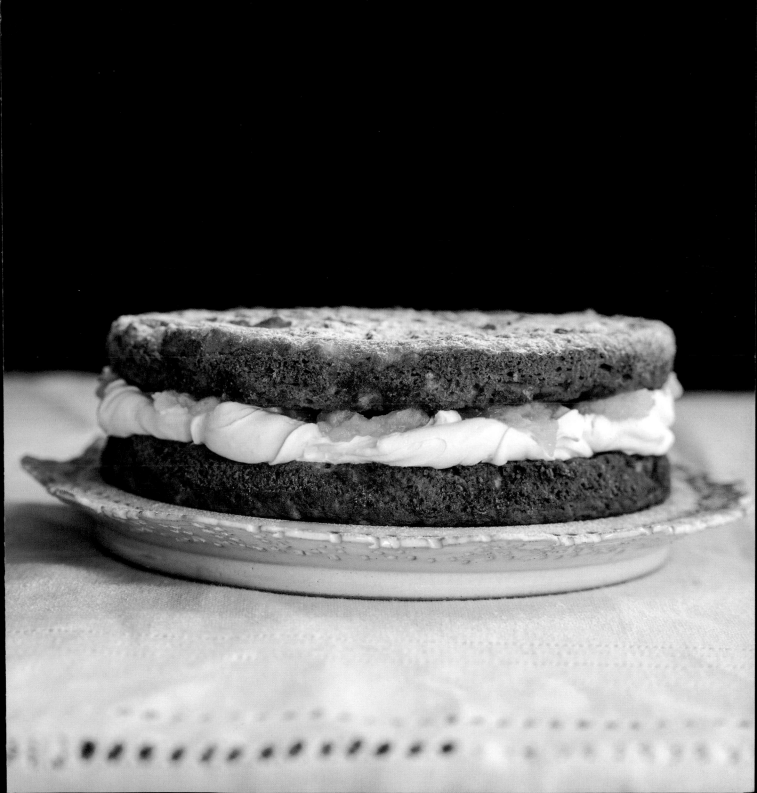

CHERRY STREUSEL CAKE

MAKES 10 SLICES

PREP: 35 MINUTES, PLUS 10 MINUTES COOLING

COOK: 1 HOUR

115g/4oz/¾ CUP RICE FLOUR
55g/2oz/½ CUP TAPIOCA FLOUR
55g/2oz/½ CUP GROUND ALMONDS
1½ TSP GLUTEN-FREE BAKING POWDER
½ TSP XANTHAN GUM
175g/6oz/¾ CUP UNSALTED BUTTER,
    AT ROOM TEMPERATURE, DICED,
    PLUS EXTRA FOR GREASING
175g/6oz/GENEROUS ¾ CUP CASTER (SUPERFINE) SUGAR
3 EGGS, BEATEN
2 TBSP SEMI-SKIMMED (LOW-FAT) MILK
½ TSP ALMOND EXTRACT (OPTIONAL)
225g/8oz FROZEN PITTED CHERRIES,
    JUST THAWED, DRAINED IF NECESSARY
GLUTEN-FREE ICING (CONFECTIONERS') SUGAR, SIFTED, TO
    DECORATE

Topping

40g/1½oz/4 TBSP RICE FLOUR
25g/1oz/¼ CUP GROUND ALMONDS
25g/1oz/2 TBSP CASTER (SUPERFINE) SUGAR
25g/1oz/2 TBSP UNSALTED BUTTER, DICED
25g/1oz/¼ CUP FLAKED (SLIVERED) ALMONDS

Cherries add a touch of summery luxury, and ready-prepared frozen cherries are becoming increasingly widely available: they need only a minute or two in the microwave on full power to thaw. Serve the cake warm with vanilla ice cream, or cold with a big spoonful of thick cream.

1. Preheat the oven to 160°C/325°F/Gas Mark 3. Butter and line the bottom of a 23cm/9in springform tin. To make the topping, put the flour, ground almonds and sugar in a bowl and mix together, then add the butter and rub in until it forms fine crumbs. Stir in the flaked almonds and set aside.

2. To make the cake, mix the flours, ground almonds, baking powder and xanthan gum together in a small bowl. Cream the butter and sugar together in a large bowl until light and fluffy, then gradually mix in the beaten eggs and flour mixture alternately, beating well between each addition. Stir in the milk and almond extract, if using.

3. Spoon the mixture into the tin and spread evenly. Spoon the cherries over the mixture, then sprinkle over the topping. Bake for about 1 hour, or until the cake is well risen, golden brown and a skewer inserted into the centre comes out clean.

4. Leave to cool in the tin for 10 minutes, then loosen the edges, remove from the tin and cool on a wire rack. Dust with icing sugar and serve. Store in the fridge in a plastic container for up to 2 days.

Cook's tip Instead of frozen cherries, you could use raspberries and diced peaches, or sliced apricots, or peeled, cored and sliced apples.

GF tip Adding ground nuts or seeds, such as flax or hulled sunflower seeds, is a good way to keep gluten-free cakes moist.

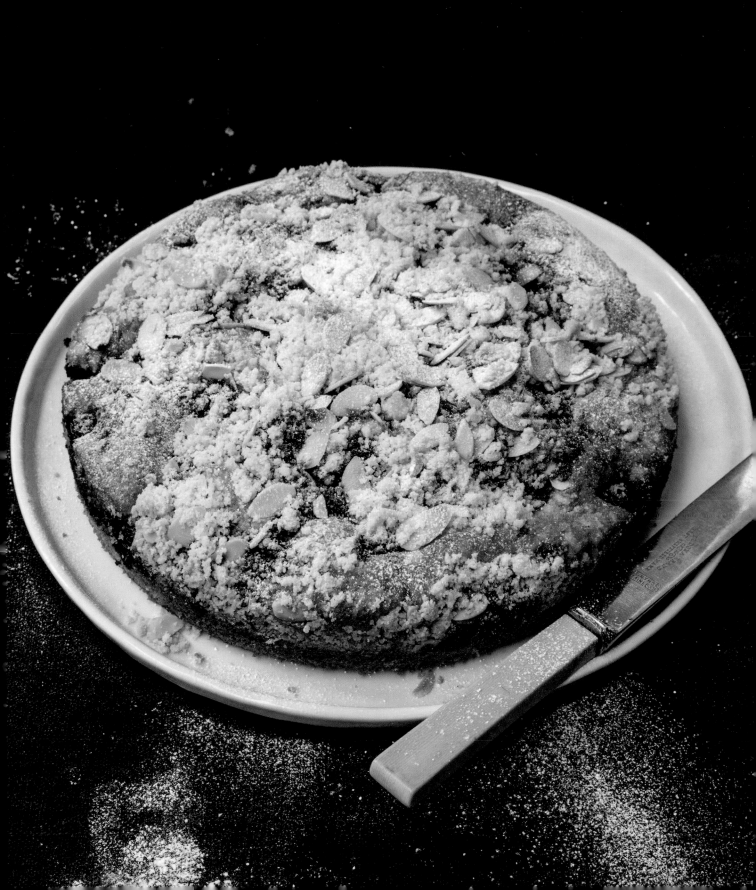

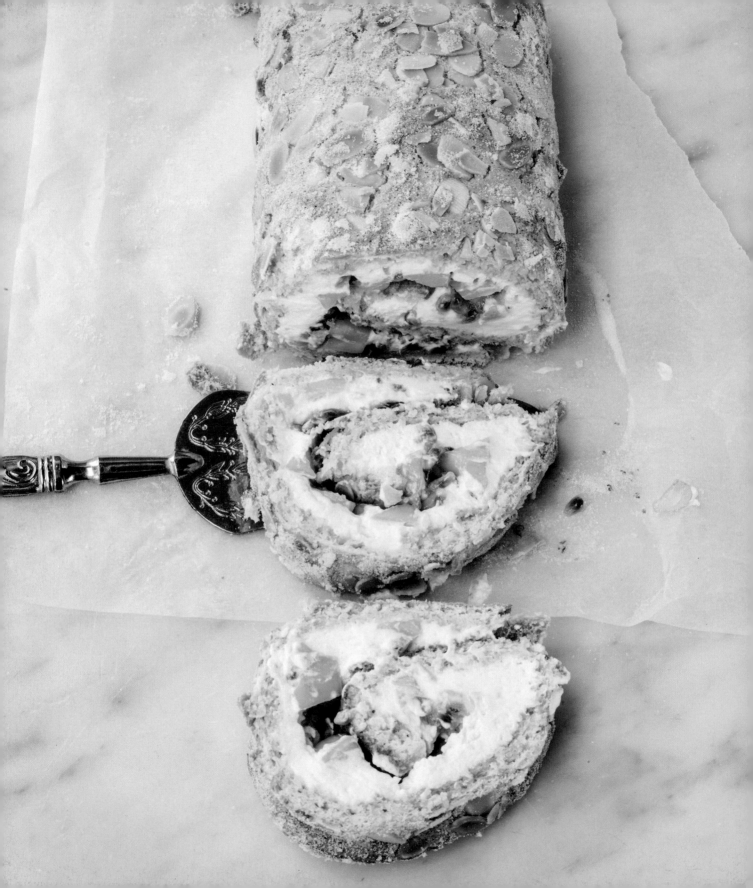

MANGO AND PASSION FRUIT ROULADE

SERVES 6
PREP: 35 MINUTES
COOK: 15–20 MINUTES

5 EGGS, SEPARATED
150g/5½oz/¾ CUP CASTER (SUPERFINE) SUGAR,
   PLUS EXTRA FOR DUSTING
100g/3½oz/1 CUP GROUND ALMONDS
3 TBSP FLAKED (SLIVERED) ALMONDS
GLUTEN-FREE ICING (CONFECTIONERS') SUGAR, SIFTED,
   TO DECORATE

Filling

1 LARGE MANGO, PITTED, PEELED AND DICED
GRATED ZEST OF 1 LIME
300ml/10fl oz/1¼ CUPS DOUBLE (HEAVY) CREAM
3 PASSION FRUIT, HALVED

Cook's tips

As there is a lot of whisking involved, this is best made with an electric whisk. If you don't have one you can speed up the whisking time by beating the egg yolks and sugar in a bowl set over a saucepan of very gently simmering water; remove from the heat while you whisk the whites.

Instead of mango and passion fruit, the cream for the filling can be flavoured with red berries, coffee or chocolate, or use cooked and puréed dried apricots, or simply spread with homemade jam.

This luxurious dessert cake is made with ground almonds. For a birthday or special occasion, decorate the top with small indoor sparklers.

1. Preheat the oven to 180°C/350°F/Gas Mark 4. Line a 23 X 33cm/9 X 13in Swiss roll tin with baking parchment and snip diagonally into the corners so that the paper lines the bottom of the tin and stands about 2.5cm/1in high around the sides.

2. Whisk the egg yolks and caster sugar together in a large bowl until very thick and pale and the whisk will leave a trail. Fold in the ground almonds.

3. Wash and dry the whisk carefully, then whisk the egg whites in a large, clean, glass bowl until soft peaks form. Fold a large spoonful into the almond mixture to loosen it, then very gently fold in the remaining egg white.

4. Spoon the mixture into the lined tin and gently ease into the corners of the tin, being careful not to knock out any air. Sprinkle with the flaked almonds and bake for 15–20 minutes, until the roulade is golden brown and springs back when lightly pressed with a fingertip. Leave to cool in the tin.

5. For the filling, mix the mango and lime zest together in a bowl, cover and set aside.

6. When ready to serve, whip the cream until it forms soft swirls. Put a large piece of baking parchment onto the work surface and dust with a little caster sugar. Turn the roulade out onto the paper with a short side nearest you. Peel off the lining paper and use a knife to mark a line about 2cm/¾in in from the short side of the roulade – this will help to give it a good shape once it is rolled.

7. Spoon the cream over the roulade, sprinkle with the mango, then scoop out the passion fruit seeds and scatter over the top. Using the paper to help, roll up the roulade from the bottom edge nearest you. Transfer to a plate, remove the paper and dust with sifted icing sugar. Cut into thick slices and serve.

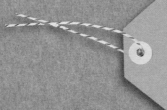

GF tip Roulades are great for those avoiding wheat flour: they can be made with ground almonds or hazelnuts, or melted chocolate.

RASPBERRY AND LEMON DRIZZLE CAKES

MAKES 8
PREP: 25 MINUTES
COOK: 18–20 MINUTES

SUNFLOWER OIL FOR GREASING
175g/6oz/¾ CUP UNSALTED BUTTER,
   AT ROOM TEMPERATURE, DICED
175g/6oz/GENEROUS ¾ CUP CASTER (SUPERFINE) SUGAR
GRATED ZEST AND JUICE OF 2 UNWAXED LEMONS
3 EGGS
175g/6oz GLUTEN-FREE WHITE SELF-RAISING
   FLOUR BLEND
3 TBSP SEMI-SKIMMED (LOW-FAT) MILK
115g/4oz/SCANT 1 CUP RASPBERRIES
150g/5½oz/¾ CUP GRANULATED SUGAR

Who can resist lemon drizzle cake? Best eaten on the day they are made, these small cakes can also be frozen: take one or two out of the freezer when you need them and add to a lunchbox or picnic basket – they will thaw in a few hours.

1. Preheat the oven to 180°C/350°F/Gas Mark 4. Grease 8 individual rectangular cake tins (10 x 5 x 3cm/4 x 2 x 1¼in or 150ml/5fl oz/⅔ cup) with a little oil and line the bottoms with a strip of baking parchment.

2. Cream the butter, caster sugar and lemon zest together in a large bowl until light and fluffy. Add one egg and beat until smooth, then mix in a little of the flour and beat until smooth. Continue adding eggs and flour alternately until all have been added, then stir in the milk to make a soft, creamy mixture.

3. Divide among the tins, spread into the corners, then press the raspberries lightly into the top of the cakes. Bake for 18–20 minutes, until the cakes are well risen, golden brown and a thin skewer inserted into the centre of a cake comes out clean.

4. Leave the cakes to cool in the tins and quickly mix the granulated sugar with the lemon juice. Spoon a little over the hot cakes, waiting until the lemon juice is absorbed before adding more. Leave to cool completely for a sugary crust to develop. To serve, loosen the edges of the cakes with a small knife, remove from the tins and peel off the paper.

Cook's tips
If you don't have little tins, some larger supermarkets now sell mini disposable loaf cases – or look online.

Instead of raspberries, you could use fresh blueberries or blackberries.

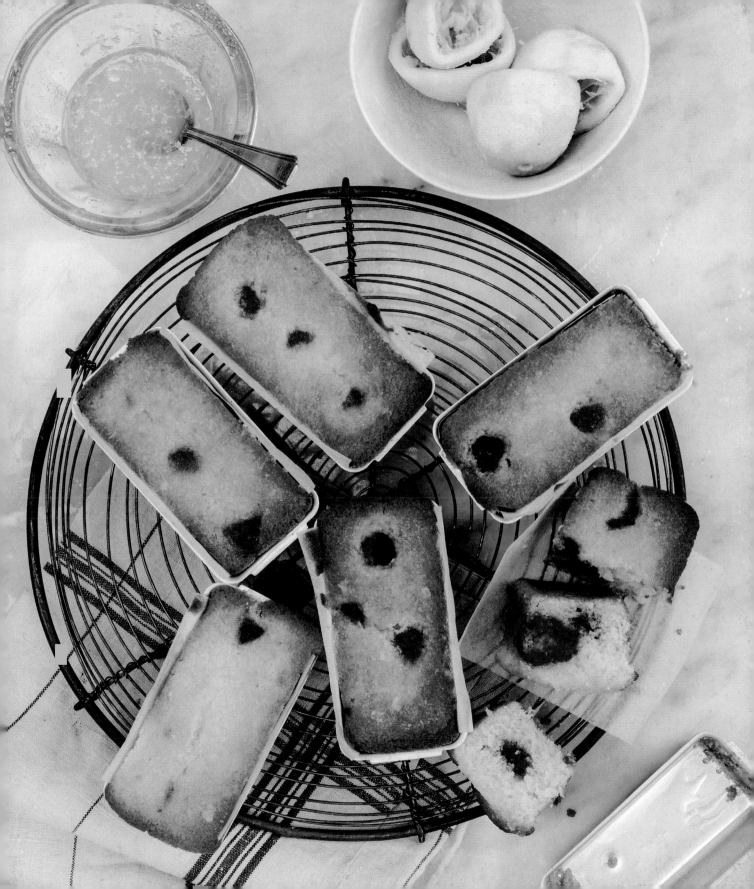

EMERGENCY MUFFINS

MAKES 12
PREP: 20 MINUTES
COOK: 15 MINUTES

175g/6oz/SCANT 1¼ CUPS RICE FLOUR
85g/3oz/SCANT ¾ CUP TAPIOCA FLOUR
150g/5½oz/¾ CUP CASTER (SUPERFINE) SUGAR
2 TSP GLUTEN-FREE BAKING POWDER
½ TSP BICARBONATE OF SODA (BAKING SODA)
½ TSP XANTHAN GUM
55g/2oz/4 TBSP UNSALTED BUTTER, MELTED
2 EGGS
200g/7oz/GENEROUS ¾ CUP LOW-FAT PLAIN YOGURT
1 TSP VANILLA EXTRACT

Flavouring

115g/4oz READY-TO-EAT DRIED APRICOTS, DICED
40g/1½oz DRIED GOJI BERRIES
2 TBSP HULLED SUNFLOWER SEEDS

If you have a large tub of natural yogurt and a few basic ingredients you can quickly fork together these muffins. They are delicious served warm straight from the oven.

1. Preheat the oven to 190°C/375°F/Gas Mark 5. Line a 12-hole muffin tin with paper cases or baking parchment.

2. Mix all the dry ingredients together in a large bowl. In a separate bowl, mix the butter, eggs, yogurt and vanilla together with a fork, then pour into the dry ingredients and fork together until only just mixed. Add the apricots and goji berries and stir briefly – the briefer the mixing, the lighter the muffins will be.

3. Spoon into the muffin cases and sprinkle with sunflower seeds. Bake for 15 minutes, until well risen, golden brown and the tops are firm when pressed with a fingertip. Cool for 10 minutes, then remove from the tin and serve while still warm.

OTHER FLAVOUR COMBOS

Leave out the apricots, goji berries and sunflower seeds and choose one of the following:

• **Double choc** – add 100g/3½oz diced gluten-free dark chocolate and 100g/3½oz diced gluten-free milk chocolate.

• **Peach melba** – add 115g/4oz fresh raspberries and 1 large stoned, diced peach.

• **Blueberry and hazelnut** – add 150g/5½oz fresh blueberries and 55g/2oz toasted and roughly chopped hazelnuts.

• **Apple and cinnamon** – grate 2 dessert apples (no need to peel) and stir in with 1 tsp ground cinnamon. Sprinkle the tops of the muffins with 2 tbsp Demerara (brown) sugar mixed with ½ tsp ground cinnamon, 1 tbsp pumpkin seeds and 1 tbsp sunflower seeds.

GF tip Baking powder sometimes includes wheat flour, so check the label before you buy. Bicarbonate of soda is not mixed with any wheat-based ingredients.

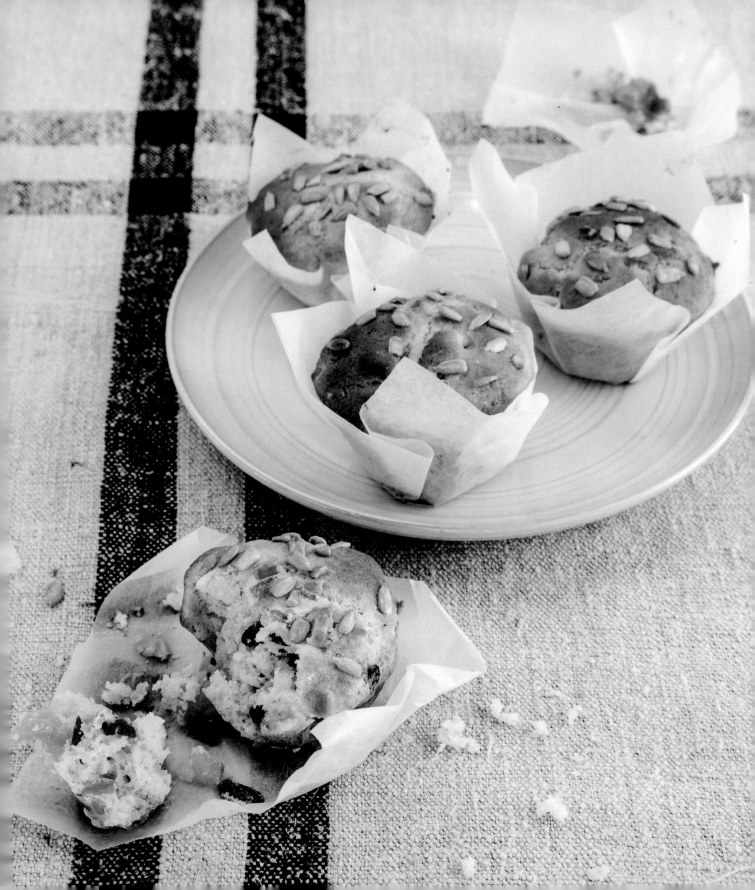

TRIPLE CHOCOLATE FINGERS

MAKES 15

PREP: 15 MINUTES, PLUS 2–3 HOURS CHILLING

55g/2oz/4 TBSP UNSALTED BUTTER

55g/2oz GLUTEN-FREE MILK CHOCOLATE, BROKEN
   INTO PIECES

85g/3oz GLUTEN-FREE DARK CHOCOLATE, BROKEN
   INTO PIECES

2 TBSP GOLDEN SYRUP

175g/6oz GLUTEN-FREE DIGESTIVE BISCUITS
   (GRAHAM CRACKERS), BROKEN INTO SMALL PIECES

100g/3½oz GLUTEN-FREE WHITE CHOCOLATE,
   BROKEN INTO PIECES

25g/1oz/3 TBSP DRIED CRANBERRIES,
   ROUGHLY CHOPPED

25g/1oz/3 TBSP PISTACHIO NUTS,
   ROUGHLY CHOPPED

55g/2oz READY-TO-EAT DRIED APRICOTS,
   ROUGHLY CHOPPED

Transform basic gluten-free digestive biscuits into something special for the kids and their friends, or to serve with coffee for the young at heart.

1. Line a 20cm/8in square shallow cake tin with a piece of baking parchment a little larger than the tin, snip the paper diagonally into the corners and press into the tin to line the bottom and sides.

2. Put the butter, milk and dark chocolate and golden syrup in a saucepan and heat very gently, stirring occasionally, until the butter and chocolate have melted and the mixture is smooth. Take the pan off the heat. Stir the biscuits into the chocolate mixture.

3. Tip the mixture into the lined tin and press into an even layer with the back of a spoon, crushing any large pieces of biscuit. Chill for 30 minutes in the fridge or 15 minutes in the freezer.

4. Melt the white chocolate in a bowl over a saucepan of gently simmering water. Drizzle over the set biscuit layer. Sprinkle the cranberries, pistachios and apricots over the top, then chill for 2 hours, until set.

5. To serve, lift out of the tin and peel away the paper. Cut into 3 bars, then cut each bar into 5 fingers. Store in the fridge for 2–3 days.

Cook's tip If you can find gluten-free chocolate buttons, use those instead of broken chocolate.

GF tip Chocolate is naturally gluten-free, but always check the label: there may be a problem with cross-contamination if the machinery is also used to make items that do contain gluten. Refer to the online directory or handbook for coeliacs so that you can choose suitable brands. Go to Coeliac UK, www.coeliac.org.uk. In the US, go to Celiac Society, www.celiacsociety.com

GF tip Gluten-free dark chocolate can taste very strong as it generally has at least 70% cocoa solids, but if you mix it with gluten-free milk chocolate you get the best of both worlds.

HONEY AND GINGER CARROT CAKES

MAKES 8

PREP: 25 MINUTES

COOK: 20 MINUTES

3 TBSP RUNNY HONEY

3 EGGS

115g/4oz/GENEROUS ½ CUP LIGHT MUSCOVADO
    (BROWN) SUGAR

150ml/5fl oz/⅔ CUP SUNFLOWER OIL

150g/5½oz CARROTS, COARSELY GRATED

40g/1½oz (2 PIECES) PRESERVED GINGER IN SYRUP,
    DRAINED AND CHOPPED

115g/4oz/¾ CUP RICE FLOUR

55g/2oz/½ CUP TAPIOCA FLOUR

1 TSP GLUTEN-FREE BAKING POWDER

1 TSP BICARBONATE OF SODA (BAKING SODA)

2 TSP GROUND GINGER

1 TSP GROUND CINNAMON

Topping

200g/7oz/¾ CUP MASCARPONE CHEESE

60g/2¼oz/½ CUP GLUTEN-FREE ICING (CONFECTIONERS')
    SUGAR

¼ TSP GROUND GINGER

1–2 SMALL PIECES OF PRESERVED GINGER IN SYRUP,
    DRAINED AND CUT INTO STRIPS

These moist, spicy, café-style cakes are perfect with a mug of good coffee or hot chocolate. Freeze any leftover cakes; thaw for 2 hours at room temperature.

1. Preheat the oven to 180°C/350°F/Gas Mark 4. Use 8 individual silicone loaf cases or small loaf tins (10 x 5 x 3cm/4 x 2 x 1¼in) – if using tins, grease and line the bottoms with a strip of baking parchment – and place on a baking sheet.

2. Put the honey, eggs, sugar and oil into a large mixing bowl and whisk together until smooth. Stir in the carrots and ginger.

3. Sift the flours, baking powder, bicarbonate of soda and spices over the carrot mixture, stir until smooth, then divide among the loaf tins. Bake for about 20 minutes, until risen, the tops feel firm and a skewer inserted into the centre comes out clean.

4. Leave to cool in the silicone cases, or loosen the edges from the metal tins and turn out onto a wire rack to cool.

5. For the topping, beat the mascarpone with the icing sugar and ground ginger, then spread over the cakes. Decorate with strips of ginger. Store in a plastic container in the fridge for up to 2 days.

Cook's tips

These moist ginger cakes can also be served without the mascarpone topping. Without the topping they will keep for 3–4 days in an airtight container.

If you don't have individual tins or silicone cases, you can bake the mixture in a small roasting pan or cake tin that measures 18 x 28cm/7 x 11in at the bottom. Bake at the same temperature for 30–35 minutes, or until the mixture springs back when pressed with a fingertip.

CHOCOLATE AND ALMOND COOKIES

MAKES 24

PREP: 20 MINUTES

COOK: 10 MINUTES

85g/3oz/6 TBSP UNSALTED BUTTER,
    AT ROOM TEMPERATURE, DICED
175g/6oz/GENEROUS ¾ CUP CASTER (SUPERFINE) SUGAR
2 TBSP UNSWEETENED COCOA POWDER
55g/2oz/6 TBSP RICE FLOUR
55g/2oz/½ CUP TAPIOCA FLOUR
1 TSP GLUTEN-FREE BAKING POWDER
1 TSP BICARBONATE OF SODA (BAKING SODA)
1 EGG
85g/3oz/GENEROUS ¾ CUP GROUND ALMONDS
100g/3½oz GLUTEN-FREE MILK CHOCOLATE, DICED
25g/1oz/¼ CUP FLAKED (SLIVERED) ALMONDS

Get the kids to help make these and eat them while still slightly warm for a wonderfully chewy, gooey texture. Or for a summer treat, sandwich with a scoop of vanilla ice cream.

1. Preheat the oven to 190°C/375°F/Gas Mark 5. Line 2 large baking sheets with baking parchment.

2. Cream the butter and sugar together in a bowl or food processor until light and fluffy. Sift the cocoa, flours, baking powder and bicarbonate of soda into the creamed mixture, add the egg and beat until smooth.

3. Stir in the ground almonds, then the diced chocolate. Spoon into 24 mounds on the baking sheets, leaving space for them to spread. Sprinkle with the flaked almonds and bake for 8–10 minutes, until the tops are cracked and a deep brown.

4. Leave to cool on the paper; serve slightly warm or leave to cool completely. Lift off the paper and store in an airtight container for 2–3 days.

Cook's tip You could replace the flaked almonds with additional diced white or dark chocolate.

GF tips

The chocolate masks the flavour of the ground almonds, but they give the biscuits a moistness that is often missing with gluten-free flours.

As these biscuits do not contain gluten they tend to go quite firm as they go cold, but after a few hours will soften again.

CHOCOLATE PEANUT BROWNIES

MAKES 24 SMALL PIECES
PREP: 25 MINUTES
COOK: 25–30 MINUTES

200g/7oz GLUTEN-FREE DARK CHOCOLATE,
    BROKEN INTO PIECES
150g/5½oz/GENEROUS ½ CUP UNSALTED BUTTER, DICED
3 EGGS
200g/7oz/1 CUP LIGHT MUSCOVADO (BROWN) SUGAR
85g/3oz/5–6 TBSP GLUTEN-FREE CRUNCHY
    PEANUT BUTTER
55g/2oz/½ CUP TAPIOCA FLOUR
1 TSP GLUTEN-FREE BAKING POWDER

Just as a brownie should be: a cracked top on a rich, moist, chocolatey base, no extra adornment needed. The peanut butter adds a delicate nuttiness and helps to keep the brownies squidgy.

1. Preheat the oven to 180°C/350°F/Gas Mark 4. Cut a sheet of baking parchment a little larger than an 18 x 28cm/7 x 11in baking tin, then snip the paper diagonally into the corners and press into the tin to line the bottom and sides.

2. Put the chocolate and butter in a bowl set over a saucepan of gently simmering water, making sure that the water doesn't touch the bottom of the bowl, and leave for 5–10 minutes, stir until smooth.

3. Meanwhile, put the eggs, sugar and peanut butter in a large bowl and beat with an electric mixer until thick and frothy. Gradually beat in the chocolate and butter mixture until smooth.

4. Mix the flour and baking powder together, then fold into the chocolate mixture. Pour into the prepared tin and ease into the corners. Bake for 25–30 minutes, until the top is crusty and slightly cracked around the edges, but still a little soft when lightly pressed with a fingertip.

5. Leave to cool in the tin, then cut into 24 pieces. Best eaten on the day, or store in an airtight container for up to 2 days.

Cook's tip The success of a brownie is all down to how long it is cooked. Ovens vary, so keep an eye on the brownies towards the end of cooking time: you want the top to look crusty but to feel almost wobbly, like a baked custard, in the centre. They will firm up as they cool. Too long in the oven and the brownies will taste dry.

GF tip Chocolate and peanut butter are not always gluten-free: it depends on the brand. The label information isn't always clear, so double-check in a recommended directory of gluten-free foods. Go to Coeliac UK, www.coeliac.org.uk. In the US, go to Celiac Society, www.celiacsociety.com

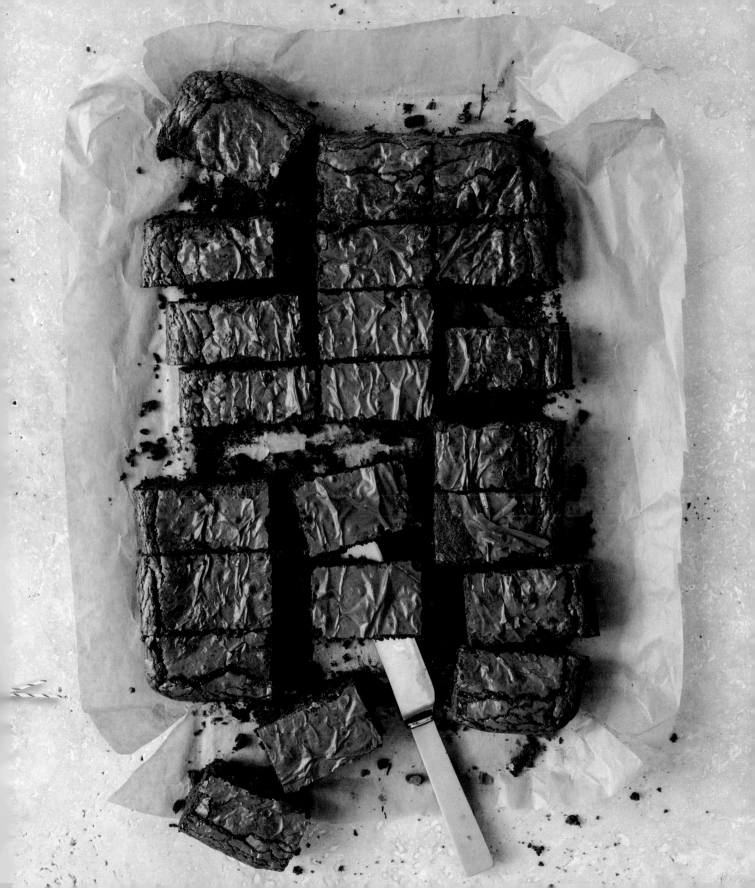

ROSEMARY AND ORANGE SHORTBREAD

MAKES 12 PIECES

PREP: 20 MINUTES

COOK: 30–35 MINUTES

55g/2oz/7 TBSP GLUTEN-FREE CORNFLOUR
    (CORNSTARCH)
115g/4oz/¾ CUP RICE FLOUR
85g/3oz/GENEROUS ¾ CUP GROUND ALMONDS
85g/3oz/SCANT ½ CUP CASTER (SUPERFINE) SUGAR,
    PLUS EXTRA FOR SPRINKLING
175g/6oz/¾ CUP UNSALTED BUTTER, AT ROOM
    TEMPERATURE, DICED
GRATED ZEST OF ½ ORANGE
1 TBSP FINELY CHOPPED FRESH ROSEMARY LEAVES

If you have a food processor the shortbread mixture can be blitzed in no time. Lovely with a cup of tea, or for dessert with a fruit fool or scoop of ice cream.

1. Preheat the oven to 160°C/325°F/Gas Mark 3. Put the cornflour and rice flour into a mixing bowl or food processor. Add the ground almonds and sugar, then add the butter and rub in or blitz until the mixture forms fine crumbs.

2. Add the orange zest and rosemary and mix until the mixture begins to stick together and form a ball.

3. Tip the mixture into a 25cm/10in loose-bottomed fluted tart tin and press evenly into the tin, using lightly wetted fingertips or the back of a fork. Mark the edge of the shortbread with the tines of a fork and prick the centre.

4. Bake for 30–35 minutes, until the shortbread is pale golden. Leave to cool in the tin for a few minutes, then mark into 12 wedges. Sprinkle with caster sugar and leave to cool completely. Remove from the tin and cut into wedges. Store in an airtight tin for 2–3 days.

Cook's tip Instead of orange, use a little grated lemon zest, or omit the orange and rosemary and add 1 tsp vanilla extract, or a few lavender petals.

GF tip Although cornflour is naturally gluten-free it may be blended with small amounts of wheat flour or processed in machinery that also mills wheat flour – always check the label.

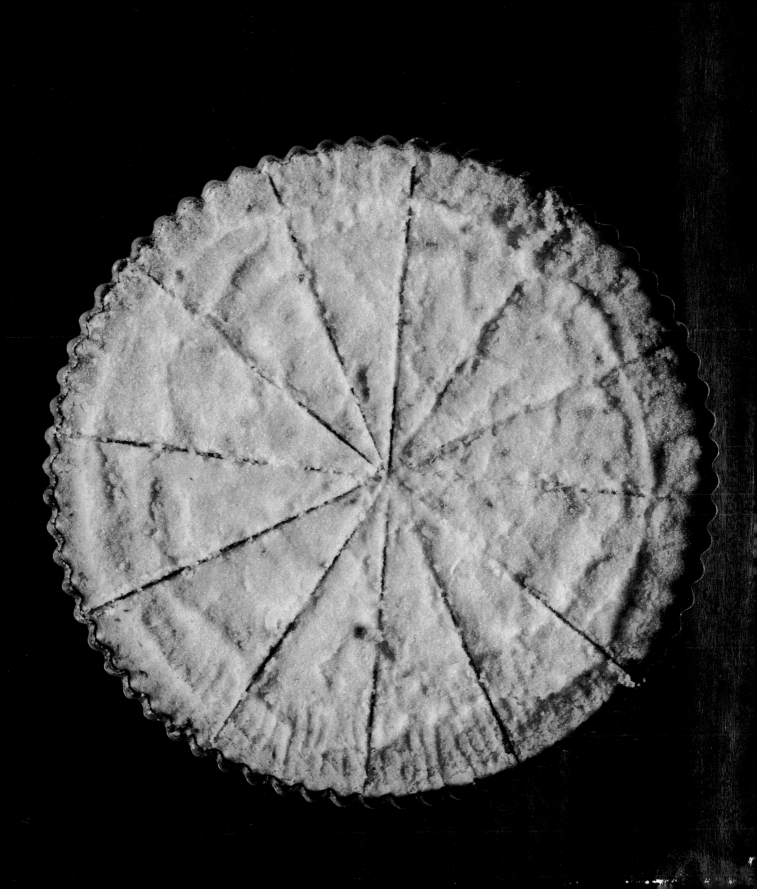

INDEX

A

allergies 8
almonds: chocolate and almond cookies 153
apples: apple and cinnamon muffins 148
  apple sauce cake 140
  cheese soufflé with cidered apples 58
  cranberry, apple and orange pie 88
  double crust blackberry and apple pie 87
  orchard pudding 125
apricots: raised pork pie 74–6
  rich fruit cake 139
  triple chocolate fingers 150
aubergines (eggplant): pastitsio 27

B

bacon: bacon and broccoli quiches 71
  bacon, leek and tarragon stuffing 56
bananas: banana, cranberry and polenta cake 138
  individual chocolate and banana pavlovas 121
  sticky tamarind and banana upside-down pudding 124
basil: pesto 24
bean sprouts: pad thai 22
beans: beetroot and black bean chilli 61
béchamel, sage 20
beef: beef carbonnade with chive dumplings 50
  beef en croûte 68–70
  bobotie 57
beer 51
  beef carbonnade with chive dumplings 50
beetroot and black bean chilli 61
bhajis, onion and cauliflower 41
biscuits: chocolate and almond cookies 153
  rosemary and orange shortbread 156
  triple chocolate fingers 150
  walnut and buckwheat thins 106
black beans: beetroot and black bean chilli 61
blackberries: double crust blackberry and apple pie 87
blueberries: blueberry and hazelnut muffins 148
  cinnamon pancakes with blueberry compote 44
  plum and blueberry pie 88
bobotie 57
bread 97–113
  coriander and cumin flatbreads 107
  date and sunflower seed soda bread 110
  pumpkin and flaxseed bread 112
  sun-dried tomato and olive focaccia 102
  techniques 100–1
broccoli: bacon and broccoli quiches 71

brownies, chocolate peanut 154
buckwheat flour: walnut and buckwheat thins 106

C

cakes: apple sauce cake 140
  banana, cranberry and polenta cake 138
  celebration chocolate cake 136
  cherry streusel cake 142
  chocolate peanut brownies 154
  honey and ginger carrot cakes 152
  mango and passion fruit roulade 145
  raspberry and lemon drizzle cakes 146
  rich fruit cake 139
  techniques 134–5
cardamom pods: chocolate and cardamom sponge puddings 128
carrot cakes, honey and ginger 152
casseroles 48
  beef carbonnade with chive dumplings 50
  lamb and chestnut cobbler 52
cauliflower: cauliflower cheese picnic pies 83
  onion and cauliflower bhajis 41
cheese: blue cheese and rocket soufflé 60
  cauliflower cheese picnic pies 83
  cheese soufflé with cidered apples 58–60
  cheesy corn muffins 104
  cheesy leek griddle cakes 43
  pastitsio 27
  pea and rocket gnocchi 24
  pecorino cheese straws 84
  pizza 108–9
  roasted red pepper and goat's cheese quiches 72
cheesecake, Florentine 118
cherry streusel cake 142
chestnuts: lamb and chestnut cobbler 52
chicken: chicken and chorizo pasta bake 29
  chicken pot pies 77–8
  raised pork pie 74–6
  roast chicken 54
  Vietnamese noodle salad 21
chickpea flour see gram flour
chillies: beetroot and black bean chilli 61
  chilli chocolate sauce 128
chive dumplings 50
chocolate: celebration chocolate cake 136
  chilli chocolate sauce 128
  chocolate and almond cookies 153
  chocolate and cardamom sponge puddings 128
  chocolate curls 92
  chocolate éclairs 122

chocolate peanut brownies 154
  double choc muffins 148
  Florentine cheesecake with Marsala peaches 118
  individual chocolate and banana pavlovas 121
  raspberry profiteroles 122
  triple chocolate fingers 150
chorizo: chicken and chorizo pasta bake 29
Christmas mince pies 94
Christmas pear and mincemeat pie 88
chutney, quick tomato and coriander 36
cider: apple sauce cake 140
  cidered apples 58
cinnamon: apple and cinnamon muffins 148
  cinnamon pancakes with blueberry compote 44
cobbler, lamb and chestnut 52
coconut: coconut custard 126
  plum, strawberry and coconut crumble 126
coeliac disease 7–8
cookies, chocolate and almond 153
coriander: coriander and cumin flatbreads 107
  coriander and ginger dip 41
  quick tomato and coriander chutney 36
  salmon and coriander fish cakes 36
corn muffins, cheesy 104
courgettes (zucchini): Mediterranean picnic pies 81
cranberries: banana, cranberry and polenta cake 138
  cranberry, apple and orange pie 88
  triple chocolate fingers 150
crème pâtissière 92
crêpes, spinach and salmon 39
cross-contamination 14
crumble, plum, strawberry and coconut 126
curry: bobotie 57
custard, coconut 126

D

dates: date and sunflower seed soda bread 110
  rich fruit cake 139
dried fruit: Christmas mince pies 94
  rich fruit cake 139
dumplings, chive 50

E

éclairs, chocolate 122
eggplant see aubergines
eggs: mustard Scotch eggs 34–5
  Vietnamese noodle salad 21
emergency muffins 148

F

fennel: individual fish pies 80
fish: individual fish pies 80
  see also salmon, sea bass etc
flatbreads, coriander and cumin 107
flaxseeds: pumpkin and flaxseed bread 112
Florentine cheesecake with Marsala peaches
  118
flours 9, 11
  for bread 98
  for cakes 132
  for pastry 64
focaccia, sun-dried tomato and olive 102
freezers 14
fries 31–45
fritto misto 40
fruit cake 139
fruit compotes 116

G

game lasagne with sage béchamel 20
garlic: garlic and red pepper sauce 40
  garlic mushroom picnic pies 83
  sun-dried tomato and garlic stuffing 56
ginger: coriander and ginger dip 41
  honey and ginger carrot cakes 152
  roasted rhubarb and ginger pavlova 120
gluten intolerance 7
gnocchi 18
  pea and rocket gnocchi 24
  sun-dried tomato gnocchi with puttanesca
  sauce 26
goat's cheese: roasted red pepper and goat's
  cheese quiches 72
gram (chickpea) flour: coriander and cumin
  flatbreads 107
griddle cakes, cheesy leek 43
guar guar gum 10

H

hazelnuts: blueberry and hazelnut muffins 148
  hazelnut and leek tart 86
honey and ginger carrot cakes 152
hot water crust pastry 74–6
hygiene 14

I

individual fish pies 80
ingredients, gluten-free 9–11

L

lamb: lamb and chestnut cobbler 52
  pastitsio 27
lasagne: game lasagne with sage béchamel 20
leeks: bacon, leek and tarragon stuffing 56
  cheesy leek griddle cakes 43
  chicken pot pies 77–8
  hazelnut and leek tart 86
lemon: lemon and herb stuffing 54
  lemon and lime tart 91

  raspberry and lemon drizzle cakes 146
limes: lemon and lime tart 91

M

mango and passion fruit roulade 145
Marsala peaches 118
mascarpone cheese: Florentine cheesecake with
  Marsala peaches 118
  honey and ginger carrot cakes 152
meatloaf: bobotie 57
Mediterranean picnic pies 81–3
meringues 116
  individual chocolate and banana pavlovas
  121
  minted pineapple pavlova 121
  roasted rhubarb and ginger pavlova 120
mile high strawberry tarts 92
mince pies, Christmas 94
mincemeat: Christmas pear and mincemeat pie
  88
minted pineapple pavlova 121
monkfish: individual fish pies 80
muffins: apple and cinnamon muffins 148
  blueberry and hazelnut muffins 148
  cheesy corn muffins 104
  double choc muffins 148
  emergency muffins 148
  peach melba muffins 148
mushrooms: beef en croûte 68–70
  chicken pot pies 77–8
  game lasagne with sage béchamel 20
  garlic mushroom picnic pies 83
  lamb and chestnut cobbler 52
mustard Scotch eggs 34–5

N

noodles 18
  pad thai 22
  Vietnamese noodle salad 21

O

oats 10
olives: onion and black olive quiches 72
  puttanesca sauce 26
  sun-dried tomato and olive focaccia 102
onions: onion and black olive quiches 72
  onion and cauliflower bhajis 41
oranges: banana, cranberry and polenta cake
  138
  cranberry, apple and orange pie 88
  rosemary and orange shortbread 156
orchard pudding 125

P

pad thai 22
pancakes, cinnamon 44
passion fruit: mango and passion fruit roulade
  145
pasta 18
  chicken and chorizo pasta bake 29

game lasagne with sage béchamel 20
  pastitsio 27
pastitsio 27
pastries: chocolate éclairs 122
  pecorino cheese straws 84
  raspberry profiteroles 122
  see also quiches; pies; tarts
pastry 63–95
  hot water crust pastry 74–6
  spinach and potato samosas 42
  techniques 66–7
pavlova: individual chocolate and banana
  pavlovas 121
  minted pineapple pavlova 121
  roasted rhubarb and ginger pavlova 120
pea and rocket gnocchi 24
peaches: Florentine cheesecake with Marsala
  peaches 118
  peach and raspberry pie 88
  peach melba muffins 148
peanut butter: chocolate peanut brownies 154
pears: Christmas pear and mincemeat pie 88
  orchard pudding 125
pecorino cheese straws 84
peppers: beetroot and black bean chilli 61
  garlic and red pepper sauce 40
  Mediterranean picnic pies 81
  pastitsio 27
  roasted red pepper and goat's cheese quiches
  72
pesto 24
picnic pies, Mediterranean 81
pies: cauliflower cheese picnic pies 83
  chicken pot pies 77–8
  Christmas mince pies 94
  Christmas pear and mincemeat pie 88
  cranberry, apple and orange pie 88
  double crust blackberry and apple pie 87
  garlic mushroom picnic pies 83
  individual fish pies 80
  Mediterranean picnic pies 81–3
  peach and raspberry pie 88
  plum and blueberry pie 88
  raised pork pie 74–6
  spinach picnic pies 83
pine nuts: pesto 24
pineapple: minted pineapple pavlova 121
pistachio nuts: triple chocolate fingers 150
pizza 108–9
plums: orchard pudding 125
  plum and blueberry pie 88
  plum, strawberry and coconut crumble 126
polenta: banana, cranberry and polenta cake
  138
  cheesy corn muffins 104
pork: mustard Scotch eggs 34–5
  raised pork pie 74–6
potatoes: extra crunchy roast potatoes 56
  individual fish pies 80
  pea and rocket gnocchi 24

salmon and coriander fish cakes 36
spinach and potato samosas 42
prawns (shrimp): pad thai 22
Vietnamese noodle salad 21
profiteroles, raspberry 122
prunes: chocolate and cardamom sponge puddings 128
puddings 115–29
pumpkin and flaxseed bread 112
pumpkin seeds: date and sunflower seed soda bread 110
puttanesca sauce 26

Q
quiches: bacon and broccoli quiches 71
onion and black olive quiches 72
roasted red pepper and goat's cheese quiches 72
see also tarts

R
raised pork pie 74–6
raspberries: peach and raspberry pie 88
peach melba muffins 148
raspberry and lemon drizzle cakes 146
raspberry profiteroles 122
rhubarb and ginger pavlova 120
rich fruit cake 139
rocket: blue cheese and rocket soufflé 60
pea and rocket gnocchi 24
rosemary and orange shortbread 156
roulade, mango and passion fruit 145

S
sage béchamel 20
salad, Vietnamese noodle 21
salmon: individual fish pies 80
salmon and coriander fish cakes 36

spinach and salmon crêpes 39
Vietnamese noodle salad 21
see also smoked salmon
samosas, spinach and potato 42
sausages: mustard Scotch eggs 35
Scotch eggs, mustard 34–5
sea bass: fritto misto 40
seafood: fritto misto 40
shortbread, rosemary and orange 156
shrimp see prawns
smoked salmon and dill soufflé 60
soda bread, date and sunflower seed 110
soufflés: blue cheese and rocket soufflé 60
cheese soufflé with cidered apples 58–60
smoked salmon and dill soufflé 60
spinach: spinach and potato samosas 42
spinach and salmon crêpes 39
spinach picnic pies 83
sponge puddings, chocolate and cardamom 128
sticky tamarind and banana upside-down pudding 124
strawberries: celebration chocolate cake 136
mile high strawberry tarts 92
plum, strawberry and coconut crumble 126
streusel cake, cherry 142
stuffings: bacon, leek and tarragon 56
lemon and herb 54
sun-dried tomato and garlic 56
sunflower seeds: date and sunflower seed soda bread 110
sweetcorn: cheesy corn muffins 104

T
tamarind and banana upside-down pudding 124
tarts: hazelnut and leek tart 86
lemon and lime tart 91

mile high strawberry tarts 92
see also quiches
tofu: Vietnamese noodle salad 21
tomatoes: beetroot and black bean chilli 61
Mediterranean picnic pies 81
pastitsio 27
pizza 108–9
quick tomato and coriander chutney 36
sun-dried tomato and garlic stuffing 56
sun-dried tomato and olive focaccia 102
sun-dried tomato gnocchi with puttanesca sauce 26
triple chocolate fingers 150
tuna: Vietnamese noodle salad 21

V
venison: game lasagne with sage béchamel 20
Vietnamese noodle salad 21

W
walnut and buckwheat thins 106
wheat allergies 8

X
xanthan gum 10, 98

Z
zucchini see courgettes